CERVICAL SPONDYLOSIS

Its early diagnosis and treatment. A book for the non-specialist and general practitioner

Cervical Spondylosis

Its early diagnosis and treatment

Edited by

Marcia Wilkinson, D.M., F.R.C.P.

Consultant Neurologist, Elizabeth Garrett Anderson Hospital and the Hackney Group of Hospitals. Director, Regional Neurological Unit, Eastern Hospital, Hackney, and Director, City Migraine Clinic.

WILLIAM HEINEMANN · MEDICAL BOOKS · LIMITED

LONDON

First Published 1967
Second Edition 1971

ISBN 0 433 36300 2

Printed by offset in Great Britain by
William Clowes and Sons, Limited, London, Beccles and Colchester

Preface to the First Edition

Cervical spondylosis was hardly recognised twenty years ago. New knowledge first took the form of clarifying its pathology and everyday symptomatology. A later development was the realisation of its possible effects on the cerebral circulation, and there has been a growing recognition of the many diagnostic difficulties to which it may give rise, and the problems of its treatment and prognosis.

Although dealing mainly with the problems of cervical spondylosis, other disorders of the cervical spine are included as their coexistence often leads to diagnostic difficulties. Radiology plays an important part in the diagnosis of congenital lesions and other abnormalities which may complicate the clinical picture. Prognosis and treatment are still matters of dispute, so having summarised conflicting views we have set out conclusions based on our own experience.

We have been very fortunate in our collaborators whose contributions speak for themselves, and we are most grateful to our publishers for their assistance, and particularly for their generosity in the matter of illustrations.

BRAIN
MARCIA WILKINSON

January 1967

Preface to the Second Edition

The late Lord Brain's untimely death just after the publication of "Cervical Spondylosis and other disorders of the Cervical Spine" was a great loss to the medical profession especially those working in the field of Neurology. "Cervical Spondylosis" was finished shortly before his death and was the last book that he completed. The present book differs from the earlier one in that much of the highly specialised anatomy has been omitted and more emphasis has been put on the early diagnosis and treatment of cervical spondylosis thus making it more useful for the non-specialist and the general practitioner.

I am most grateful to my collaborators for their contribution and to the publishers for their constant help and assistance.

December 1970 — MARCIA WILKINSON

List of Contributors

Ruth E. M. Bowden, D.Sc., M.B., B.S.(Lond.), M.R.C.S.(Eng.)
Professor of Anatomy, Royal Free Hospital School of Medicine, University of London; Hunterian Professor of the Royal College of Surgeons of England.

Geoffrey O. Storey, M.D., M.R.C.P., D.Phys.Med.
Consultant in Rheumatology and Physical Medicine, Hackney Group of Hospitals.

Lindsay Symon, T.D., F.R.C.S.
Consultant Neurosurgeon, The National Hospitals for Nervous Diseases, Queen Square and Maida Vale and St. Thomas's Hospital, London; Member External Scientific Staff, Medical Research Council.

Marcia Wilkinson, D.M., F.R.C.P.
Consultant Neurologist, Elizabeth Garrett Anderson Hospital and the Hackney Group of Hospitals; Director, Regional Neurological Unit, Eastern Hospital, Hackney, E.9 and Director, City Migraine Clinic, 11–12 St. Bartholomew Close, E.C.1.

Allan C. Young, M.B., B.S., D.M.R.D.
Director, Radiodiagnostic Department, St. Mark's Hospital, London.

Contents

Chapter I

Historical Introduction

MARCIA WILKINSON

Cervical spondylosis is a condition in which there is a progressive degeneration of the intervertebral discs leading to changes in the surrounding structures especially the bones and meninges. In the past this condition has been called osteoarthritis, cervical spondylitis, herniated disc, chondroma, etc., but the term spondylosis is considered preferable as the condition is a degenerative rather than inflammatory or neoplastic one.

Although it has been known for many years that lesions of the cervical spine may cause paraplegia, it was not until fairly recently that the importance of cervical spondylosis in the production of both root and cord symptoms was recognised. The first recorded reference to paraplegia following an injury to the cervical spine is found in the Edwin Smith Papyrus (Breasted, 1930) written 4,000 years ago. In this the surgeon describes five cases of injury to the cervical spine and in one he comments briefly on the condition—"One having a dislocation in a vertebra of his neck while he is unconscious of his two legs and his two arms and his urine dribbles—an ailment not to be treated." It is not known whether or not Sir Walter Raleigh had any symptoms of cervical spondylosis, but he had changes in his cervical spine which nowadays would probably be called spondylotic. John Aubrey in his *Brief Lives* says that Sir Walter Raleigh's son, Carew, had "digged up his father's grave" and that "his skull and neck-bone being viewed, they found the bone of his neck lapped over so that he could not have been hanged".

James Parkinson (1817) was interested in disorders of the cervical spine, as he thought that the symptoms of Parkinsonism were due to "a diseased state of the medulla spinalis in that part which is contained in the canal, formed by the superior cervical vertebrae, and extending, as the disease proceeds, to the medulla oblongata". Parkinson's theory of the basic pathology of parkinsonism is very interesting as we now know that compression of the vertebral artery in the spinal canal may cause ischaemic lesions of the brain stem and parkinsonism may sometimes develop. Parkinson also recognised that the cervical spine was particularly susceptible to trauma as he says "the great degree of mobility in that portion of the spine which is formed by the superior cervical vertebrae, must render it, and the contained parts, liable to injury from sudden distortions". He was obviously familiar with cases of cervical spondylosis as he goes on to describe a patient "subject to rheumatic affection of the deltoid muscle (who) had felt the usual inconvenience from it for 2 or 3 days; but at night found that the pain had extended down the arm, along the inside of the fore-arm, and on the sides of the fingers, in which a continual tingling was felt. The pain, without being intense, was such as effectually to prevent sleep; and seemed to follow the course of the brachial nerve." This is a very good account of the symptoms which occur when a cervical root is compressed, and the treatment this patient received is interesting. "Blood was taken from the back part of the neck by cupping; hot fomentations were applied for about the space of one hour, when the upper part of the back of the neck was covered with a blister.—On the following day the pains were much diminished, and in the course of 4 or 5 days were quite removed. The hand and arm now felt more than ordinarily heavy, and were evidently much weakened; aching and feeling extremely wearied after the least exertion. The strength of the arm was not completely recovered at the end of more than 12 months."

Key (1838) in his paper on paraplegia described 2 cases of spinal cord compression where "the obstruction was found to be occasioned by a projection of the intervertebral substance, or rather the posterior ligament of the spine, which was thickened, and presented a firm ridge, which had lessened the diameter of the canal by nearly a third. When the vertebrae had been divided longitudinally by the saw, the ligament, where it passes over the posterior surface of the intervertebral substance, was found to be ossified nearly throughout the whole of its fibres, and considerably increased in density." This is a particularly good description of the pathological lesion which is found in all patients with spondylosis and is probably the first description of a spondylotic bar. In this patient the lesion was probably in the upper thoracic region. Although lesions of the cervical cord had been diagnosed earlier, it was not until 1892 that the first successful operation on the cervical spine for spondylosis was done by Horsley (Taylor and Collier, 1901). At operation the cord was found to be compressed by a transverse ridge projecting backwards from the body of the vertebra. The patient was a 20-year old builder who, while under the influence of alcohol, fell off his van on to the road striking his right shoulder. He picked himself up and walked home, a distance of 300 yards. The following morning he was unable to move his right arm because of pain. Two weeks later the pain became more severe and his arms became powerless. Over the next 2 months he gradually lost control of his legs and sphincters. On October 24th, 1892, Horsley performed a laminectomy of the 6th cervical vertebra. The leptomeninges were adherent to the theca and "a transverse ridge of bone projected backwards from the body of the vertebra and pressed upon the cord". By November 3rd there was a marked improvement in movement in the arms and legs and following the operation he was free of pain. By June 1893 he was able to walk and he was reported as having completely recovered by September that year.

Gowers (1892) under the heading "Vertebral Exotoses" described exotoses growing from the bodies of the vertebrae into the spinal canal which might compress the cord or nerves. He said that they were exceedingly rare and that their chief characteristic was extreme chronicity. The symptoms might be those of slow compressions of the cord, or of irritation, expressed chiefly by pain. Gowers concluded that exostoses constituted a more promising field for the surgeon than other kinds of vertebral tumour. Many of them were so placed that their removal was feasible and if situated in front of the cord, the division of some nerve roots, at least in the dorsal region, might permit access to the growth. Gowers also alluded to the involvement of the cervical spine in chronic rheumatoid arthritis. The cord, he said was hardly ever compressed, but the narrowing of the foramina might damage the nerve roots.

Bailey and Casamajor (1911) discussed osteoarthritis of the spine as a cause of compression of the spinal cord and its roots and reported five cases. In none of these was the cervical cord involved. They noted that osteoarthritis of the spinal column was extremely common in persons past middle-age, and suggested that the primary pathological change was thinning of the intervertebral discs. They further suggested that this led to changes in the bodies of the vertebrae including bony overgrowth. They thought that these exostoses were situated at first anteriorly and laterally, and later posteriorly, and they pointed out that these posterior exostoses may compress the cord.

Elliot (1926) was perhaps the first person after Gowers to describe how spinal arthritis involving the cervical region might give rise to radicular symptoms through narrowing of the intervertebral foramina. Stookey (1928) attributed compression of the spinal cord to ventral extradural chondromas. He divided these into three groups: (1) those causing pressure on the ventral part of one half of the spinal cord, (2) those compressing both halves ventrally, and (3) those placed more laterally and so causing root compression. This was a considerable advance because so far, though involvement of nerve roots had been attributed to the osteoarthritis, the lesions producing compression of the spinal cord had been regarded as chondromas, that is to say the essentially benign nature of the lesion had not been recognised. It was Schmorl (1929), Schmorl and Junghanns (1932) and Andrae (1929) who first described the anatomical and pathological aspects of intervertebral disc protrusion from the spinal column. About the same time Beadle (1931) discussed the normal and abnormal anatomy of the intervertebral disc in relation to certain spinal deformities. In spite of the work of these authors, the concept of the chondroma persisted for some time. Kortzeborn (1930) reported the case of a patient with pains in the shoulders and arms, weakness of the right leg and difficulty in walking, who died 24 hours after operation and at autopsy was found to have a "chondroma" the size of a bean which appeared to come from the posterior aspect of the intervertebral disc between the 6th and 7th cervical vertebrae, and had compressed the spinal cord. Elsberg (1928) in a paper on extradural tumours mentioned that 7 out of 46 were "chondromas" arising from intervertebral discs, and in a later paper he reported 15 cases of "chondroma" or "echondrosis" of which 9 were in the cervical region. He noted that the prominence formed by the growth was usually a little to one or other side of the midline, though it might extend transversely from one side to the other. Bucy (1930) described 16 cases of "chondroma" of intervertebral discs of which 9 were in the cervical region.

Keyes and Compere (1932) discussed the embryology, physiology and pathology of the intervertebral disc and Peet and Echols (1932) were the first to suggest that the lesion which had hitherto been called a "chondroma" or "ecchondrosis" was really a protrusion of the intervertebral disc itself. They reported two cases of herniation of the nucleus pulposus, one of which compressed the cervical cord. Microscopically they found that the lesion consisted of a few cartilage cells, scattered throughout a relatively acellular matrix, in fact a normal nucleus pulposus with nothing to suggest either inflammation or neoplasm.

Over the next 15 years the various clinical syndromes that could arise as a result of spondylosis were described. Nachlas (1934) first drew attention to the fact that pain in the chest could result from lesions involving the cervical spine and Hanflig (1936) in discussing cervical spondylitis as a cause of pain in the shoulder and arm referred to pain in the chest wall as an associated symptom. Love and Walsh (1940) estimated that about 4 per cent of all disc lesions were in the cervical region and Stookey (1940) in a further paper on cervical disc lesions, pointed out that protrusion of cervical intervertebral discs occurred chiefly in males in later middle life, the average age in his series being 53. He distinguished three clinical pictures: first, the syndrome of bilateral ventral pressure on the spinal cord, indistinguishable from compression by a tumour in the same position; second, unilateral ventral pressure tending to produce a Brown–Séquard syndrome; and third, nerve root pressure. Semmes and Murphey (1943), and Bucy and Chenault (1944), also discussed the production of radicular symptoms by the acute protrusion of a cervical intervertebral disc. They pointed out that the pain of acute cervical disc protrusion might be accompanied by dyspnoea and closely simulate the pain of coronary occlusion. Elliott and Kremer (1945) reported further cases of protrusion of the cervical intervertebral disc and drew attention to the value of myelography in diagnosis. Spurling and Scoville (1944) reported 12 verified cases of ruptured cervical intervertebral disc; they thought that the dorsal protrusion was usually the result of trauma and tended to cause cord compression, while lateral protrusions were usually the result of degeneration and caused pain in the shoulders and upper limbs resulting from root compression. Bradford and Spurling (1945) emphasised the importance of manometry of the cerebro-spinal fluid. They demonstrated a complete block in one-third of their cases, a partial block in one-third and no abnormality in the other third. The majority of their cases had signs of cord compression. They thought that the poor results obtained from operation in the cases with compression of the spinal cord were due to the existence of irreversible changes in the anterior part of the spinal cord which had been produced by repeated trauma and which occurred with movements of the neck. Bull (1948) correlated the anatomy of the joints of the cervical spine with the mode of production of the symptoms caused by their disease and their abnormal radiological appearances. He drew attention to the importance of the neurocentral joint of Luschka, and pointed out that the presence of osteophytes invading the intervertebral foramen did not necessarily mean pressure on the nerve, and conversely the absence of osteophytes did not exclude pressure on the nerve, which might be due to swollen periarticular tissues which would not cause changes in plain X-rays. Brain (1948) discussed the importance of vascular factors as a cause of disturbance in the functions of the cervical cord for some segments below the site of compression. He drew a distinction between acute cervical disc protrusion, often traumatic in origin and more likely to compress the nerve roots than the spinal cord, and chronic protrusion associated with osteophytic outgrowths. This type of protrusion was more likely to cause cord compression. In 1948 Barnes discussed protrusion of intervertebral discs as a result of injuries to the cervical spine and drew attention to the group of patients in whom damage to the spinal cord was produced by hyperextension of the neck in a patient who already had spondylotic changes. Kaplan and Kennedy (1950) studied the effect of head posture on the manometrics of the cerebro-spinal fluid in cervical lesions. They found that changes in head posture, particularly extension during jugular compression might cause "intermittency" of spinal subarachnoid block. "Intermittency" was found in 12 patients with cervical spondylosis who had normal fluid dynamics with the head in the neutral position, and was not found in 253 patients with neurological disorders without suspicion of cord compression. They argued that the intermittency was probably due to the fact that when spondylotic protrusions were present cord compression tended to be maximal in extension and therefore a partial block was most likely to be found when the head was extended.

In 1951 Frykholm published a detailed study of patients with cervical root compression and this included a comprehensive review of the various aspects of degeneration of the intervertebral discs. In his monograph he distinguished two main types of disc protrusion, nuclear herniation and annular protrusion. The first type was due to the extrusion of nuclear material through a tear in the annulus and the second type resulted from bulging of the annulus. In both types the size of the initial protrusion might gradually increase with the addition of new tissue. A nuclear herniation is originally soft, but may be transformed into a fibrous or cartilagenous mass in which calcification may occur. An annular protrusion is usually fibro-cartilagenous but may gradually become calcified. Frykholm suggested the following classification of disc protrusion:

1. **Dorsal protrusions.** These are entirely intraspinal and emerge from the main part of the disc. They may be (a) dorsomedial, capable of producing bilateral cord compression, (b) paramedian, capable of producing unilateral cord compression, and (c) dorsolateral, capable of compressing the nerve roots intraspinally against the lateral part of the vertebral lamina.

2. **Intraforaminal protrusions.** These come from the uncinate part of the disc and compress the radicular nerve against the articular processes.

3. **Lateral protrusions.** These also come from the uncinate part of the disc and are capable of compressing the vertebral artery and veins.

4. **Ventral protrusions.** These come from the ventral margins of the disc.

Frykholm pointed out that two or more of these types are often combined. He also pointed out the main pathological lesion responsible for radicular symptoms was root-sleeve fibrosis. This is characterised by thickening and opacity of the dural root-sleeve, and adjacent parts of the dural sac, and is accompanied by thickening and fibrosis of the arachnoid membrane in the vicinity of the root ostia. This root-sleeve fibrosis is sometimes sufficient in itself to cause nerve root compression. Brain, Northfield and Wilkinson (1952) described 45 patients with spondylosis of whom 38 had compression of the spinal cord and 7 compression of the nerve roots only. They thought that the primary lesion was degeneration of the intervertebral discs and that the changes in the bodies and neurocentral joints were secondary to these. They drew a distinction between the more acute lesions involving mainly the nucleus pulposus which were usually the result of acute trauma, and the more slowly developing cervical spondylosis in which the protrusion consisted not only of the nucleus pulposus but also associated changes in the ligaments, bones and joints. Symonds (1953) described the inter-relation of trauma and cervical spondylosis in compression of the spinal cord and discussed possible mechanisms. He divided his cases into three groups, those with accidental injury added to pre-existing cervical spondylosis, those who had sudden paralysis without injury and, lastly, those who had cervical spondylosis and in whom injury had been inflicted upon the cervical spine by hyperextension during operation for some unrelated condition. He drew attention to the fact that in patients in whom compression of the spinal cord was gradual and the disability mild, the signs were frequently confined to the lower limbs with symptoms and signs extending no higher than the upper thoracic level. Mair and Druckman (1953) discussed the pathology of spinal cord lesions and considered that the changes in the spinal cord resulted from compression of the anterior spinal artery and its branches by the protruding disc as the injury principally involved the anterior horns, the lateral columns and the anterior part of the dorsal columns. Taylor (1953) thought that in cervical spondylosis the spinal cord was compressed not only by the disc protrusion but also by the ligamenta flava. He considered that these might cause recurring trauma to a cervical cord raised upon a disc protrusion or an osteophytic bar. Pallis, Jones and Spillane (1954) stressed the fact that cervical spondylosis was a common disease of elderly people. They found that 50 per cent of people over the age of 50 and 75 per cent of people over the age of 65, had typical radiological changes of cervical spondylosis; 40 per cent of people over 50 had some limitation of their neck movements and 60 per cent had some neurological abnormality. O'Connell (1955) distinguished three types of lesion occurring in cervical spondylosis. First, an intervertebral disc protrusion which is a space-occupying lesion, lying within the spinal canal and composed of intervertebral disc tissue, either annulus fibrosus or nucleus pulposus alone or a combination of both. Secondly a "primary spondylosis" in which there are degenerative changes of unknown causation and in which the joints between the vertebral bodies and the zygapophyseal joints are involved. The changes are frequently not only severe but widespread. In this type the arthritic vertebral margins separated by degenerative disc tissue form ridges across the floor of the spinal canal. Thirdly he recognised "secondary spondylosis" in which changes develop in an intervertebral joint when there is a disc protrusion and therefore localised to a single level. The abnormalities consist of a narrowing of the intervertebral disc between the vertebral bodies, sclerosis of the surfaces of these bodies adjacent to the affected discs and lipping of their margins. O'Connell thought that the neurological deficit was out of proportion to the size of the lesion as compared with a meningioma or a neuro-fibroma in a similar region and that the intervertebral disc protrusion not only compressed the spinal cord but also traumatised it with the production of irreversible changes. A disc protrusion developed more rapidly, and being harder than a neoplasm, did not accommodate itself to the available space, but severely distorted the cord, all the more, probably because the protrusion occupied only a small part of the length of the spinal canal. The extradural position of the protrusion added to the risk of cord trauma since, during movements of the spine, the mass would remain fixed whereas an intradural neoplasm moved with the theca and the cord. Clarke and Robinson (1956) analysed the case notes of 120 patients in whom spinal cord compression was due to cervical spondylosis and found that on the whole the results of treatment were disappointing. They recommended that immobilisation of the neck should first be tried and laminectomy with section of the dentate ligament should only be done if deterioration continued in spite of conservative treatment. Payne and Spillane (1957) carried out an anatomical and pathological study of the cervical spines of 70 patients. They found that in patients with myelopathy due to cervical spondylosis the average measurement of the cervical canal from C4 to C7 was smaller by about 3 mm than the standard measurement. Spondylotic changes reduced the size of the canal but myelopathy was more likely to occur when the original dimensions were smaller than normal. They also thought that the so-called joints of Luschka "were no more than unco-vertebral fissures in the lateral parts of the cervical discs". In cervical spondylosis considerable alterations took place in the shape and texture of the vertebral bodies, and defects in the cartilage plates allowed nuclear displacements into the cancellous tissues of the bodies of the adjacent vertebrae. When the disc was narrowed the resulting approximation of the bodies of adjacent vertebrae led to deformity of the uncus, marginal lipping, partial occlusion of the intravertebral foramina and ridge formation on the anterior wall of the spinal canal. Herniation of disc tissue through the annulus was commonly associated with these changes. Cervical nerves were found to be kinked or compressed as a result of changes taking place in the neighbourhood of the intravertebral foramina. Bradshaw (1957) discussed and analysed the clinical features of 78 patients with cervical spondylosis who had a neurological deficit, and stressed the difficulties of diagnosis. He found that patients with focal myelopathy improved or remained unchanged when treated with a collar; that those with generalised spondylosis most often deteriorated, and that the majority of patients with brachialgia obtained relief within days or weeks of assuming a collar. The short-term results were satisfactory, but over half the patients with myelopathy deteriorated after 6 to 18 months. Few patients with a history longer than one year made a significant recovery when a mechanical cause was found for brachialgia. If such a mechanical cause was corrected at operation at an earlier stage, relief from pain was the rule. If none was found amelioration was uncommon. Wilkinson (1960) carried out a pathological anatomical study of the cervical spine, spinal cord and nerve roots in 17 patients with cervical spondylosis who came to autopsy. She found that the primary lesion appeared to be a degeneration of the intravertebral disc and that the changes in the bodies and vertebra and neurocentral joints were secondary to this. Changes were found in the annulus fibrosus, the vertebrae and in the region of the intervertebral foramen as well as in the nucleus pulposus. These, in turn, might cause lesions of the spinal cord and nerve roots.

Taylor (1964) considered that in less than half the cases die the neurological level of dysfunction correspond to the level of the main bony lesions seen on the X-ray films and that at operation the spinal cord was seldom found to be compressed. From this he deduced that the origin of the spinal cord disorder was not direct neuronal compression but vascular insufficiency caused by arterial or venous obstruction or both.

James (1965) found that in general, the outcome in cervical spondylosis was independent of age, sex, trauma, the extent of degenerative changes, the type of clinical picture and extent of initial disability, but did depend on the duration of symptoms before diagnosis and the level of protein in the cerebrospinal fluid. He thought therefore that cervical spondylosis could produce two types of change in the spinal cord: firstly, an acute "exudative" and potentially reversible condition and, secondly, a process of gradual loss of neural tissue with subsequent demyelination and gliosis. The factor that prevents the former from progressing inevitably to the latter may be the development of a collateral circulation.

Hughes (1966) in a prospective series of 200 consecutive adult necropsies found 15 patients with myelopathy and 6 with radiculopathy due to cervical spondylosis. He considered that "the narrowing of the anteroposterior diameter of the spinal canal produced by the spondylotic protrusions transcended in importance any other single finding". Hughes and Brownell (1964) reported one case where there was occlusion of the anterior spinal artery due to cervical spondylosis and they comment that this is a very rare finding. Recent observations on the effect of cervical spondylosis on the cerebral circulation are described elsewhere.

References

Andrae, R. (1929), *Beitr. path. Anat.*, **82**, 464.
Aubrey, J. (1949), *Brief Lives*, edited by Anthony Powell, London.
Bailey, P. and Casamajor, L. (1911), *J. nerv. ment. Dis.*, **38**, 588.
Barnes, R. (1948), *J. Bone Jt. Surg.*, **30B**, 234.
Beadle, O.A. (1931), "The Intervertebral Disc", *Spec. Rep. Ser. med. Res. Counc., Lond.*, No. 161.
Bradford, F. K., and Spurling, R. G. (1945), *The Intervertebral Disc*, 2nd edition, Thomas, Springfield, Ill., p. 121.
Bradshaw, P. (1957), *Quart. J. Med.*, **26**, 177.
Brain, W. R. (1948), *Proc. R. Soc. Med.*, **41**, 509.
Brain, W. R., Northfield, D. W. C. and Wilkinson, M. (1952), *Brain*, **75**, 187.
Breasted, J. H. (1930), *The Edwin Smith Surgical Papyrus*, Chicago, Vol. 1.
Bucy, P. C. (1930), *J. Amer. med. Ass.*, **94**, 1552.
Bucy, P. C. and Chenault, H. (1944), *J. Amer. med. Ass.*, **126**, 26.
Bull, J. W. D. (1948), *Proc. R. Soc. Med.*, **41**, 513.
Clarke, E. and Robinson, P.K. (1956), *Brain*, **79**, 483.
Elliott, F. A. and Kremer, M. (1945), *Lancet*, **i**, 4.
Elliott, G. R. (1926), *J. Bone Jt. Surg.*, **8**, 42.
Elsberg, C. A. (1928), *Surg. Gynec. Obstet.*, **46**, 1.
Elsberg, C. A. (1931), *Bull. neurol. Inst., N.Y.*, **i**, 350.
Frykholm, R. (1951), *Acta chir. scand.*, suppl. 160.
Gowers, W. R. (1892), *Diseases of the Nervous System*, 2nd edition, Vol. 1, Churchill, London, p. 260.
Hanflig, S. S. (1936), *J. Amer. med. Ass.*, **106**, 523.

Hughes, J. T. and Brownell, B. (1964), *Neurology, Minneap.*, **14**, 1073.
Hughes, J. T. (1966), *Pathology of the Spinal Cord*, Lloyd Luke, London.
James, J. L. (1965), "The Treatment of Myelopathy due to Cervical Spondylosis", MD Thesis, Bristol University.
Kaplan, L. and Kennedy, F. (1950), *Brain*, **73**, 337.
Key, C. A. (1838), *Guy's Hosp. Rep.*, **3**, 17.
Keyes, D. C. and Compere, E. L. (1932), *J. Bone Jt. Surg.*, **14**, 897.
Kortzeborn, A. (1930), *Abl. Chir.*, **57**, 2418.
Love, J. G. and Walsh, M. N. (1940), *Arch. Surg.*, **40**, 454.
Mair, W. G. P. and Druckman, R. (1953), *Brain*, **76**, 70.
Mixter, W. J. and Ayer, J. B. (1935), *New Engl. J. Med.*, **213**, 385.
Nachlas, I. W. (1934), *J. Amer. med. Ass.*, **103**, 323.
O'Connell, J. E. A. (1955), *Brit. J. Surg.*, **43**, 225.
Pallis, C. A., Jones, A. M. and Spillane, J. D. (1954), *Brain*, **77**, 274.
Parkinson, J. (1817), An essay on the Shaking Palsy, London.
Payne, E. E. and Spillane, J. D. (1957), *Brain*, **80**, 571.
Peet, M. M. and Echols, D. H. (1932), *Arch. Neurol. Psychiat., Chicago*, **32**, 924.
Schmorl, G. (1929), *Fortschr. Röntgenstr.*, **40**, 18.
Schmorl, G. and Junghanns, H. (1932), *Die gesunde und kranke Wirbelsäule im Röntgenbild; pathologisch-anatomische. Untersuchingen*, Thieme, Leipzig.
Semmes, R. E. and Murphey, F. (1943), *J. Amer. med. Ass.*, **121**, 1209.
Spurling, R. G. and Scoville, W. B. (1944), *Surg. Gynec. Obstet.*, **78**, 350.
Stookey, B. (1928), *Arch. Neurol. Psychiat., Chicago*, **20**, 275.
Stookey, B. (1940), *Arch. Surg.*, **40**, 417.
Symonds, C. P. (1953), *Lancet*, **i**, 451.
Taylor, A. R. (1953) *Lancet*, **i**, 717.
Taylor, A. R. (1964), *Neurology, Minneap.*, **14**, 62.
Taylor, J. and Collier, J. (1901), *Brain*, **24**, 532.
Wilkinson, M. (1960), *Brain*, **83**, 589.

Chapter II

The Applied Anatomy of the Cervical Spine

RUTH E. M. BOWDEN

The cervical spine is only one part of a single, versatile and complex organ which has regional variations in structure, function and vulnerability to injury and disease. This part of the vertebral column supports and moves the head; provides attachment for muscles suspending and moving the upper limb girdles and for some respiratory muscles.

The transverse processes of the upper six cervical vertebrae transmit the vertebral arteries and surrounding venous plexuses. These vessels provide the main blood supply of the medulla, pons, cerebellum and visual cortex, and the spinal cord. Segmental branches and tributaries not only supply vertebral joints, but also the roots of the cervical and brachial plexuses, the spinal nerves from which they are derived, the meninges, and more centrally, they anastomose with the longitudinal channels of the spinal vessels.

The marrow in the bodies of the lower six cervical vertebrae, in common with that of other regions, is haemopoeitic throughout life, and therefore subject to metastatic deposits.

THE CERVICAL VERTEBRAE AND ARTICULATIONS

The shapes of the vertebrae and their alignment are seen from anterior, lateral and posterior views in Figures 2.1, 2.2 and 2.3 respectively. The cervical lordosis (Fig. 2.2) develops late in foetal life and increases when the baby first lifts his head and again when he sits up. This curve, which is due to wedging of intervertebral discs, begins in the upper thoracic region and the convexity is at its maximum in the region of joints between the 4th and 5th cervical vertebrae (Fig. 2.4).

The head is balanced on the oval, concave articular facets on the upper surface of the atlas, and the head and atlas move as one when rotating round the odontoid peg. Three series of joints form columns which support and move the head. In the mid-line anteriorly there are the cartilagenous joints between the bodies of the vertebrae (Figs. 2.1 and 2.2) and more laterally and posteriorly there are the right and left synovial joints between the laminae (Figs. 2.2 and 2.3). The total surface area of these zygapophyseal joints is approximately two-thirds of the articular area between the bodies (Davis, personal communication). The joints between the 7th cervical and 1st thoracic vertebrae mark a transition between a highly mobile and a less mobile region of the spine. The laminae of the 7th rest on a shelf on the 1st thoracic vertebra. This prevents downward movement (Davis and Rowland, 1965) and may contribute to certain types of whip-lash injury of the neck, since the most mobile part of the lower cervical spine is close to this, between the 5th and 6th vertebrae.

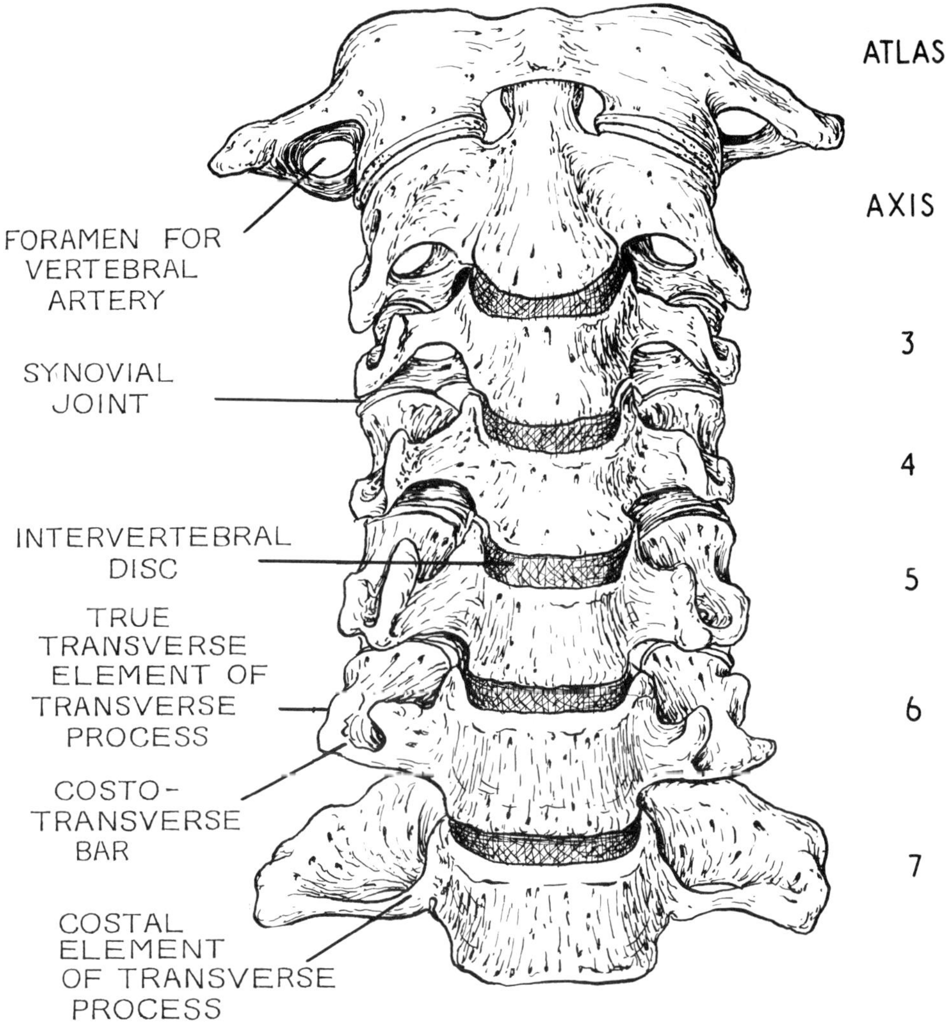

Fig. 2.1 Anterior view of articulated cervical vertebrae

The joints

The shape and mode of articulation of the joints influences the axes and possible ranges of movement, and in every case the form of the articular surfaces is more complicated than appears in the articulated cervical column (Figs. 2.1, 2.2 and 2.3).

(a) Those between the bodies of the lower 6th cervical and the 1st thoracic vertebra are concave-convex. In dried specimens the upper vertebra tends to override the lower. The upper surfaces of the 3rd cervical to the 1st thoracic vertebrae have

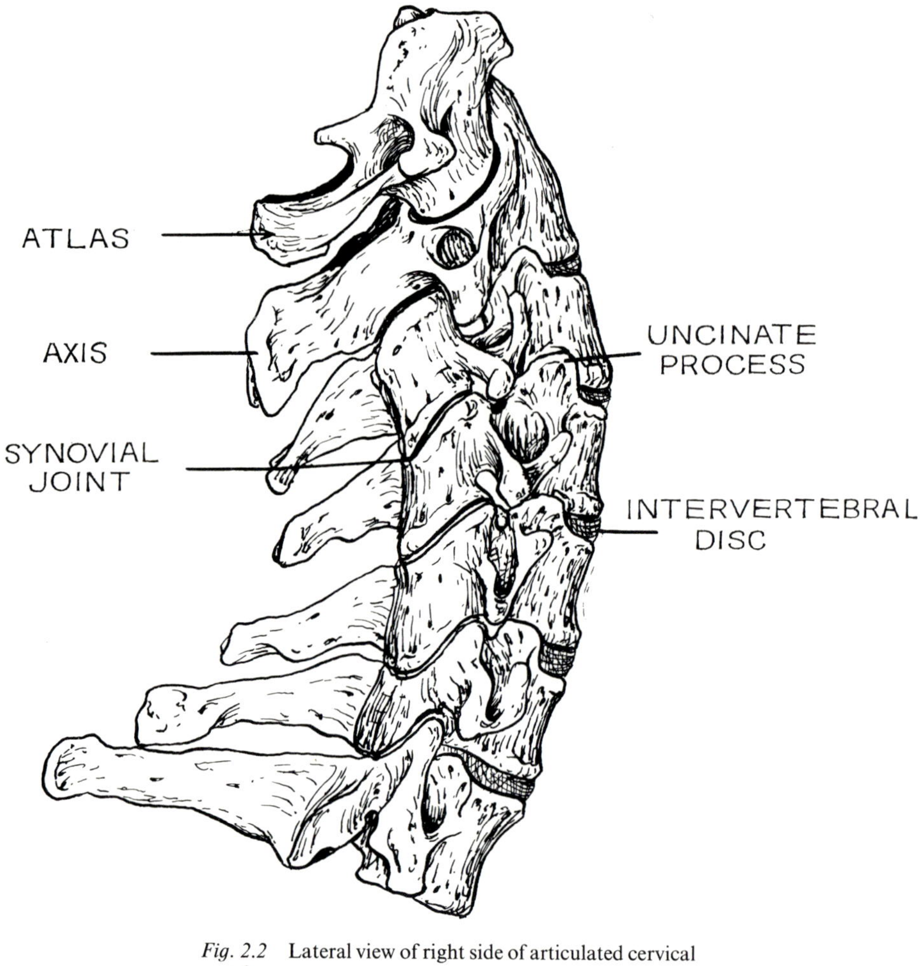

Fig. 2.2 Lateral view of right side of articulated cervical vertebrae

small uncinate processes at the anterior boundary of the intervertebral foramina. The articular surfaces of the bodies are covered with plates of avascular hyaline cartilage and they are united by intervertebral discs. These discs increase in area from below the axis downwards and the cervical lordosis is produced by their wedged shape. The thickness of the discs varies, the two deepest lie below the

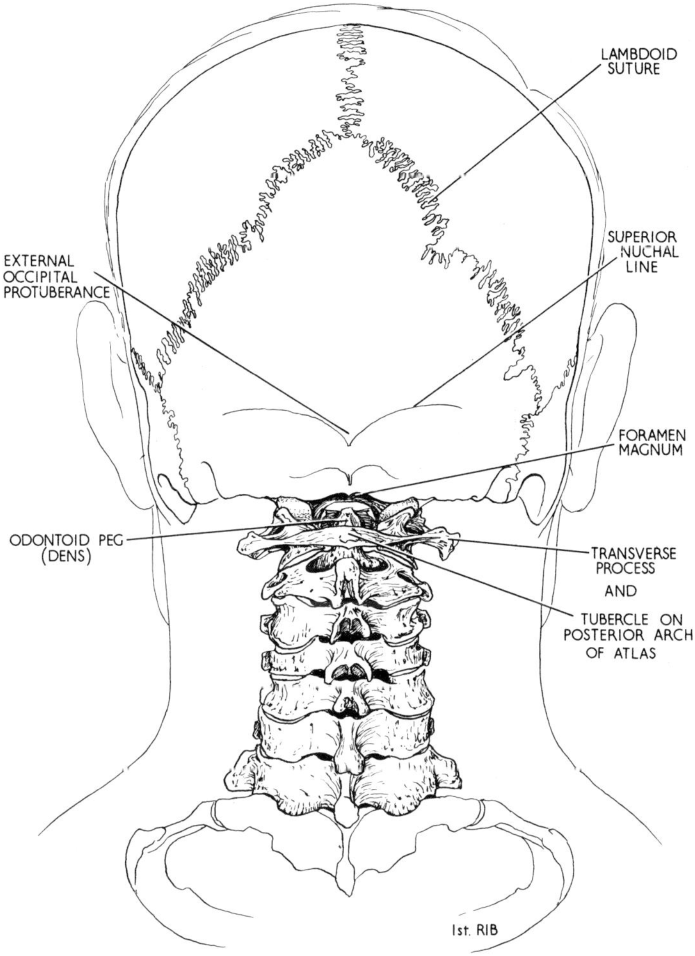

Fig. 2.3 Posterior view of skull, cervical vertebrae, first thoracic vertebra and first ribs

sixth and fifth vertebrae respectively (Todd and Pyle, 1928). Each disc is formed of fibrocartilage and contains a nucleus pulposus which is a remnant of the embryonic notocord. The nucleus is deformable but incompressible. It is held under pressure by the obliquely and concentrically arranged fibres of the disc which are attached to a ring of compact bone on the margins of vertebral bodies. The nucleus is nearer the spinal canal than the anterior surface of the vertebral bodies. The latter increase in girth

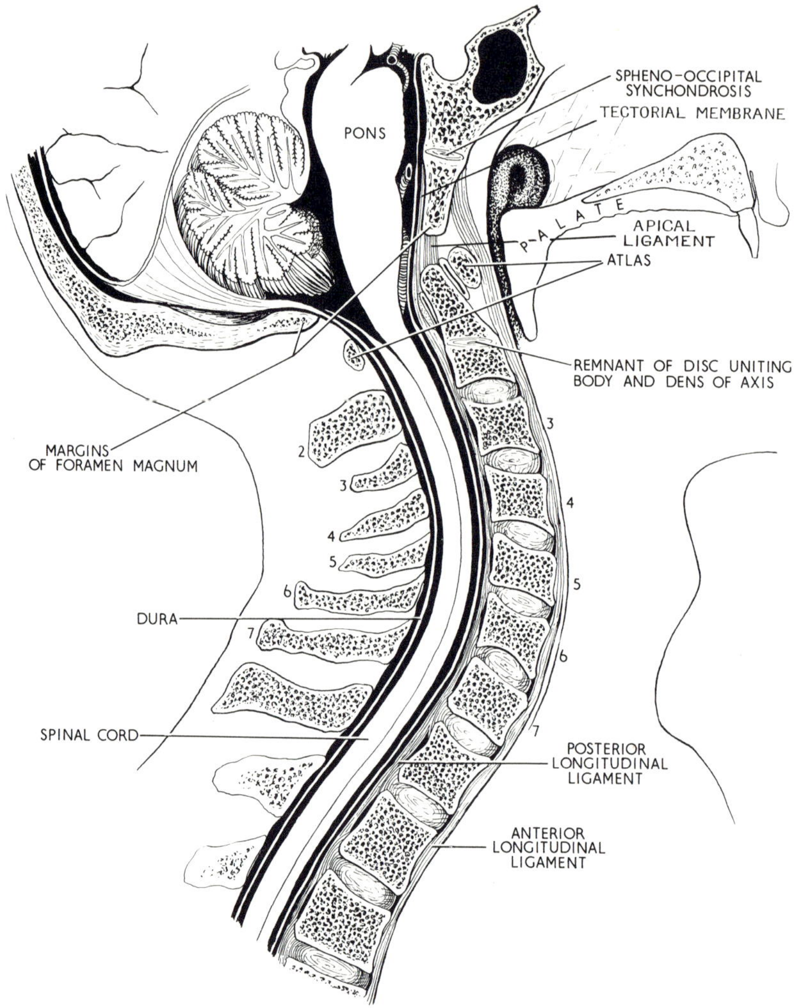

Fig. 2.4 Midline section of the head and neck to show the relations of the dura, spinal cord and hind brain to the bones, ligaments and joints between the bodies of the vertebrae. Note the cervical lordosis; the relations of the anterior and posterior longitudinal ligaments to the intervertebral discs; and the ligaments at the cranio-vertebral junction

during development and growth by deposition of bone on the front and sides, whilst the spinal canal is increasing in diameter.

In the cervical region small bursa-like cavities develop during childhood in the discs where they impinge on the uncinate processes. These are not true synovial joints, but for all practical purposes may be considered as such because of their function and their reaction to degenerative and traumatic processes. The existence of these uncovertebral joints has been disputed and the evidence is reviewed by Penning (1968).

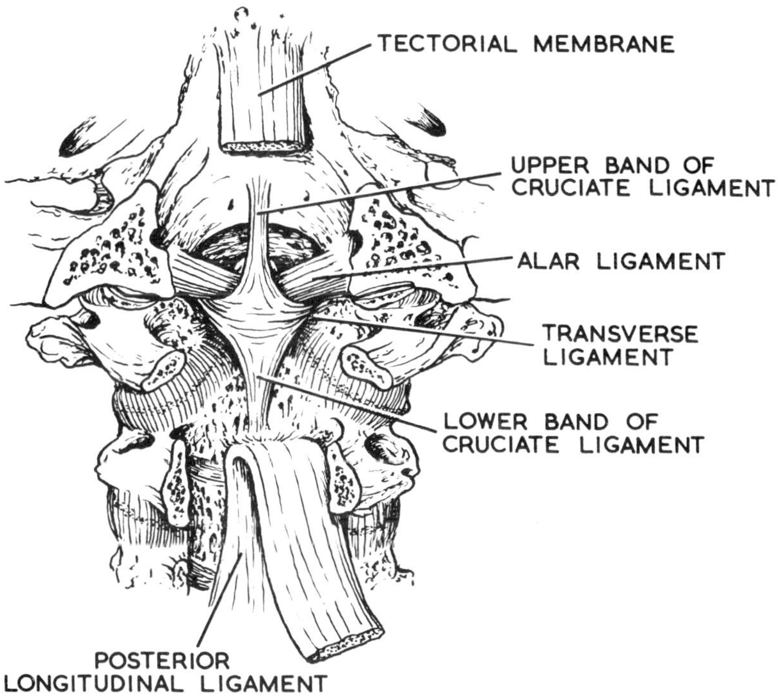

Fig. 2.5 Ligaments of the cranio-vertebral joints seen from behind with the posterior longitudinal ligament (tectorial membrane) cut and turned down

The vertebral bodies are also joined by anterior and posterior longitudinal ligaments which extend up to the occipital bone and down into the sacrum. The anterior ligament is firmly fixed to the bodies and is so lightly fixed at the discs that a sudden, but not necessarily violent, extending force may rupture it and lead to a severe hyperextension associated with irreversible damage to the spinal cord (O'Connell, 1955; Stoltmann and Blackwood, 1964). The posterior ligament is very firmly fixed to the discs and adjacent bones, but not to the centre of bodies where the vessels enter and leave the marrow cavity (Fig. 2.4).

(b) The articular surfaces of the synovial joints are covered with avascular hyaline cartilage, which is dependent upon underlying bone and synovial fluid for its maintenance. The capsules of the joints are relatively small in area compared with the articular surface and efficient blood supply is particularly important.

The atlanto-occipital and atlanto-axial joints are specialised and are controlled by highly innervated intersegmental muscles. The elongated and convex occipital condyles roll backwards and forwards in the reciprocally concave facets on the upper surface of the atlas.

The head and atlas move as one around the odontoid peg and the upper articular facets of the axis. The long transverse processes of the atlas provide the arms of the levers used in rotation (Figs. 2.1 and 2.3). The anterior surface of the odontoid articulates with the posterior surface of the anterior arch of the atlas. The peg is anchored by alar ligaments and by the apical ligament, a fibrous continuation and remnant of the notocord (Figs. 2.4 and 2.5). It rotates in front of a small transverse ligament from which it is separated by a bursa. The cruciate ligaments and the prolongation of the posterior longitudinal ligament cover over the odontoid and its restraining ligaments and are attached above the anterior lip of the foramen magnum inside the posterior cranial fossa. In this region the posterior longitudinal ligament is known as the tectorial membrane (Figs. 2.4 and 2.5). The obliquely directed postero-lateral joints (Figs. 2.1 and 2.2) allow the atlas to rotate on the axis with a downward screwing movement.

The remaining synovial joints are oval or circular in outline and are curved in cross section. The concavities and convexities are not necessarily congruous or symmetrical. These joints, combined with those between the bodies permit flexion, extension, a measure of rotation and lateral flexion. Virtually all movements and particularly lateral flexion are associated with some rotation.

Analysis of Movements of the Cervical Spine

Although the total excursion of the head in flexion, extension, rotation and lateral flexion can be measured, it is exceedingly difficult to analyse the ranges of movement at any particular joint. The techniques involve highly sophisticated radiology and meticulous measurements and these have been reported and reviewed recently by Penning (1968). The overall range of movement in the sagittal plane (flexion and extension) is given as 90° by O'Connell (1945) and 80·5° by Bakke (1931), about three-quarters being due to extension. Approximately 10° of flexion and 25° of extension occur at the atlanto-occipital joints (Fielding, 1957; Penning, 1968). Fielding also reported about 5° of flexion and 10° of extension at the atlanto-axial joints, Penning (1968) gave a larger range. This unexpected finding of sagittal movement at the atlanto-axial joints underlines the importance of the ligaments in protecting the spinal cord from damage by the normal, fractured or dislocated odontoid process (McRae, 1960).

The remainder of the full range in this plane is contributed by the lower parts of the cervical spine. The maximum range of movement between individual vertebrae is at the level of the joints between the 4th and 5th vertebrae in young children and between the 5th and 6th in teenagers (Zeitler and Markuske, 1962). In adults the most mobile joint lies at the latter level (Breig, 1960; Davis, 1960; Penning, 1961), where one of the two thickest intervertebral discs is found.

In flexion, the anterior parts of an intervertebral disc are compressed and the incompressible nucleus pulposus tends to be shifted backwards if there is any weakness or damage to the annulus fibrosus. The annulus is stretched posteriorly, the intervertebral foramina are widened (Frykholm, 1951) and the spinal canal is lengthened more posteriorly than anteriorly (Breig, 1960) but in general it is straightened out (Penning and Van der Zwaag, 1966). In extension, the annulus fibrosus tends to bulge into the spinal canal, the intervertebral foramina are narrowed and the stout elastic ligamenta flava that unite the laminae of neighbouring vertebrae also tend to bulge into the canal.

The total range of rotation of the head and neck is estimated to be about 80–90°. About 35–45° occurs at the atlanto-axial joint and this is associated with a screwing movement of the upper on the lower bone, a movement which reduces the cross-sectional area of the spinal canal.

Lateral flexion does not occur in isolation but is accompanied by some rotation. Werne (1957) reported a total range of 4° to 13·5° of lateral flexion at the atlanto-occipital joint. Penning (1968) found about 30° of lateral mobility on both sides in the lower cervical spine. The spinal canal is shortened on the side of the concavity of the spine and lengthened on the side of the convexity.

Changes in the Joints Due to Age or Degeneration

The intervertebral disc and nucleus pulposus undergo daily reversible changes which result in slight shortening of the total length of the spinal column (de Puky, 1935). It is suggested that this is due either to dehydration or to the persistence of a tract for the notocord into which the nucleus pulposus may be forced by movements and weight bearing. In addition there are biochemical changes, increasing fibrosis and progressive dehydration in both the fibrocartilage of the discs and the nucleus pulposus and both may even become calcified. They become more vulnerable to chronic and acute trauma. With loss of disc substance, the annulus fibrosus may bulge into the spinal canal, and on account of its eccentric position the nucleus tends to prolapse backwards if there is any tear in the annulus. The commonest sites for both types of herniation are at the most mobile regions, namely at C5–6 and C6–7 (Bull, 1951; Mixter, 1951). A persistent track for the notocord may lead to a central herniation. The nucleus may expand and compress the vertebral bodies as in young patients (Schmorl's disease) and in senile osteoporosis (Beadle, 1931; Coventry, Ghormley and Kernohan, 1945a–c).

In all these conditions there is a narrowing of the disc space, and shortening of the length of the spinal column. The intervertebral foramina are narrowed, movements are restricted and unusual mechanical strains are imposed on the synovial joints.

These changes may be confined to a localised area or be widespread in generalised degenerative changes. The formation of osteophytes may lead to encroachment upon the spinal canal and intervertebral foramina (Fig. 2.6). The canal may also be further narrowed by bulging of the ligamenta flava.

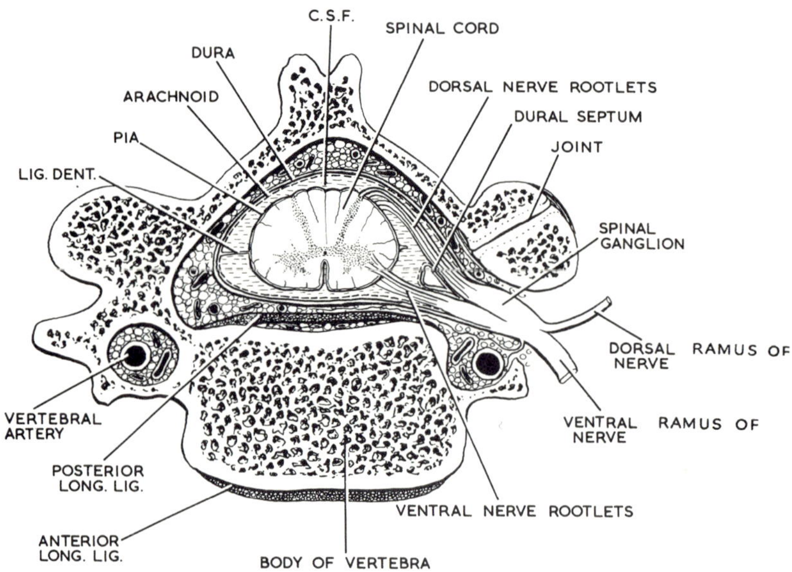

Fig. 2.6 Relations of dura to bone and roots of nerve shown in an oblique transverse section. On the right the relations between the emergent nerve and the synovial joint are seen, but the joint between the vertebral bodies is not in the plane of section

The degenerative changes in the joints may be exacerbated by distortion of the vertebral artery due to shortening of the column (Fig. 2.7), especially if there are associated plaques in the walls of the vessel. Branches supplying joints and nervous tissue are distorted at rest and further obstructed with movement. On occasion the ischaemia may be so severe that syncope results from rotation of the head (Biemond, 1951; Hutchinson and Yates, 1956). Chronic relative ischaemia leads to a vicious circle of degenerative changes in bones, synovial membranes and joints. One of the most serious complications of damage to the cervical spine is the effect upon the related spinal cord, nerve roots and meninges (Frykholm, 1951a–d; Brain, Northfield and Wilkinson, 1952; Abdullah and Bowden, 1960).

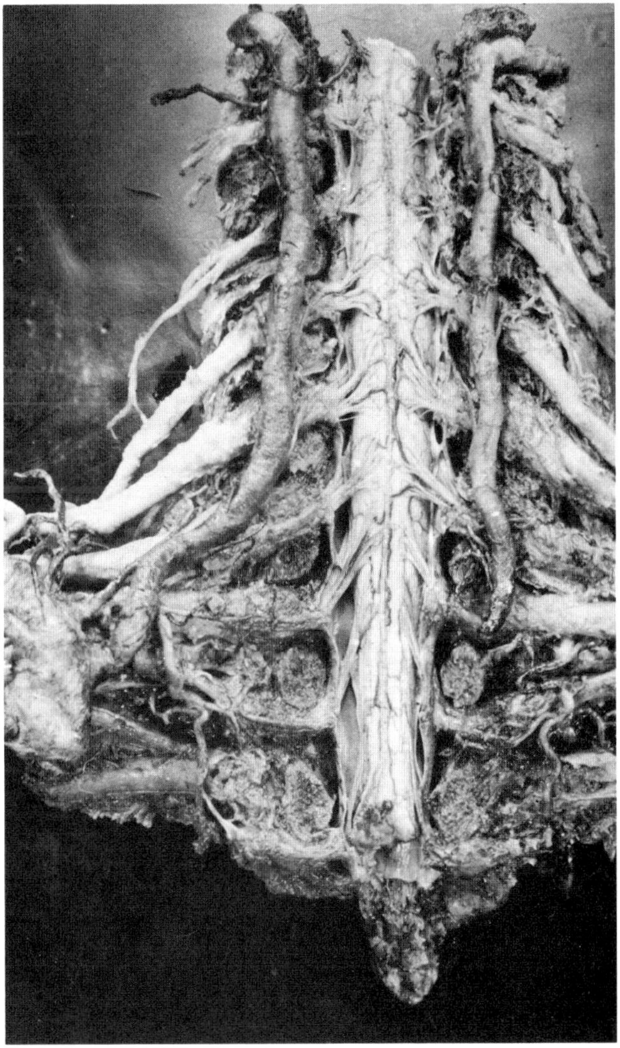

Fig. 2.7 Note the early changes in the vertebral artery after shortening of the vertebral canal by degeneration of intervertebral discs (Dissection by S. Abdullah)

THE RELATIONS OF THE MENINGES, SPINAL CORD AND NERVE ROOTS TO THE CERVICAL VERTEBRAE

The inner layer of the dura mater is continued as a sac from the posterior cranial fossa (Fig. 2.4) down to the second, third or fourth sacral vertebra. It is tethered above to the margins of the foramen magnum and below by the filum terminals which continues from the end of the cord through the theca to the coccyx. Laterally the sleeves of dura which transmit dorsal and ventral roots of spinal nerves, the spinal nerves and

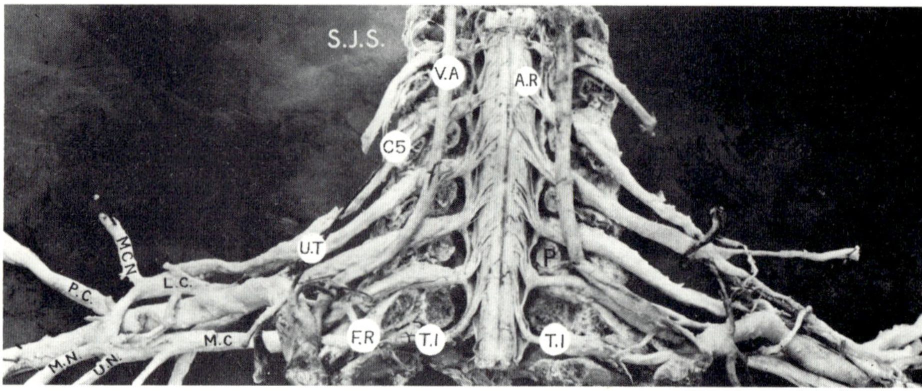

Fig. 2.8 Spinal cord, membranes, vessels, anterior rootlets of spinal nerves with symmetrically formed brachial plexuses *in situ*.

Anterior view, Case 15, female aged 64 years (Abdullah)

- A.R. = anterior rootlets
- C5 = fifth cervical nerve
- F.R. = first rib
- Tl = first thoracic nerve
- U.T. = upper trunk of brachial plexus
- L.C. = lateral, M.C. = medial, P.C. = posterior: cords of plexus
- M.C.N. = musculo-cutaneous nerve
- M.N. = median nerve
- U.N. = ulnar nerve
- V.A. = right vertebral artery. Note the relationship of the artery to the nerves and ganglia
- P = left pedicle of the seventh cervical vertebra, with the eighth cervical nerve inferior to it
- S.J.S. = right synovial joint space between third and fourth cervical vertebrae

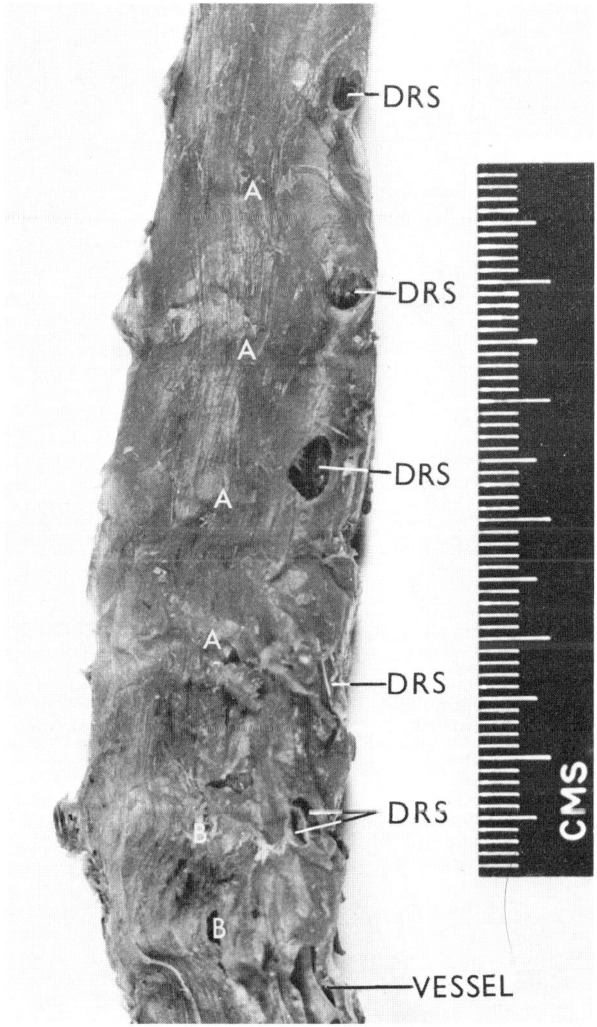

Fig. 2.9 Specimen from dissecting room of 92 year old female. Indentations (A) on the anterior surface of the dural sac due to hypertrophic degenerative changes in bodies of vertebrae at the level of the intervertebral discs.

Note: the relationship of these to the opened dural root sleeves (DRS). The lowest sleeve shows dorsal and ventral compartments. B. the tears in the dura made on separation from the densely adherent posterior longitudinal ligament accompanying vessels, are lightly attached to the margins of the intervertebral foramina. Anteriorly the dura is firmly attached to the margins of the intervertebral foramina. Posteriorly the dura is firmly attached to the posterior ligament behind the upper two cervical vertebrae, and thereafter only lightly fixed to the ligament. It has no posterior attachments.

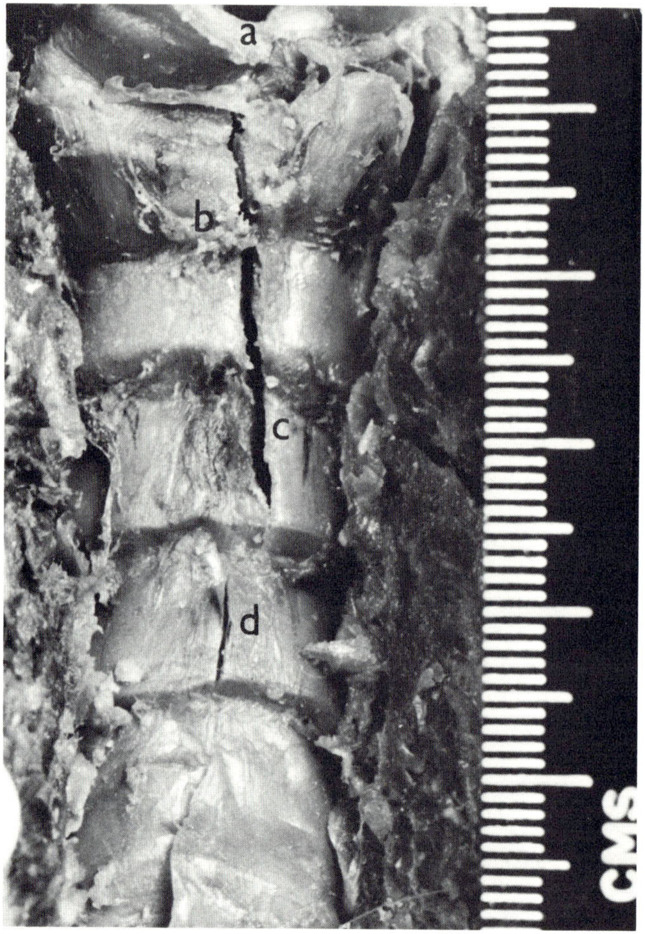

Fig. 2.10 The posterior view of the dura *in situ* showing concertina like folds of dura mater

a = atlas b = adhesions

Note the thickness of the dura which had been opened at c and d

Early in foetal life the spinal cord is co-extensive with the spinal canal, but the column grows more rapidly than the cord. By birth the lower end of the latter is at the lower border of the third lumbar vertebra and by 3 years in most individuals it reaches its definitive level opposite the disc between the first and second lumbar vertebrae. In some it may be lower and in others higher than this level. In consequence, there is an increasing obliquity of nerve roots passing from the cord to the appropriate ostia of the dural sleeve and increasing angulation of the sleeves and nerves at the intervertebral foramina. The rootlets of the cervical and upper thoracic nerves are shown in Figure 2.8 in the neutral position. Movements of the spine affect the dura, arachnoid, pia and the contained nervous tissues. Even movements of the lower limb which are associated with movements of the lumbar spine produce some traction on the cervical nerve roots and possibly the cord.

Flexion decreases the angle between the lower border of the dural root sleeve and the dural sac, it also decreases the angulation of the rootlets of the nerve as they enter the dorsal and ventral openings into the single dural root sleeve. The dura and spinal cord are stretched dorsally. In extension the converse occurs, and angulation of rootlets of nerves increases at the dural ostia. Lateral flexion to the left stretches the nerve roots on the right, slackens those on the left, the root sleeves converge on the left and diverge on the right. Rotation produces differential tensions on the anterior and posterior rootlets of a single nerve. Turning the chin to the right stretches the right dural sleeve and the right dorsal rootlets and slackens the ventral ones; on the left the sleeve and dorsal rootlets slacken and the ventral rootlets are stretched.

The rootlets, the dorsal root ganglia, common spinal nerves and their extrinsic and intrinsic blood vessels are held in a firm dural sleeve, which is in turn attached to the margins of the intervertebral foramen. Should there be any narrowing of the foramen or any adhesions due to past trauma, extension and rotation might lead to further cumulative congestion, oedema and compression of the nerves and their vessels (Frykholm, 1951d). [The extrinsic and intrinsic vessels of the cervical spinal cord, nerve rootlets and roots are described elsewhere (Bowden, Abdullah and Gooding, 1967).] In theory rotation might also lead to damage by tearing capillaries and it is regrettable that this was the one movement which was not restricted in the multicentral trial of treatment of pain in the neck (Brewerton, 1966).

Since the membranes and neural structures are so intimately related to the vertebrae and their joints (Fig. 2.8) they may be distorted and damaged by changes in the latter and/or by the accompanying obstructions to the blood vessels. Figures 2.9–11a and b show the changes found in a dissecting room specimen taken from a woman of 92 years. Unfortunately, no history is available. There was a marked senile kyphosis of the thoracic spine, with an increased compensatory lordosis of the neck. Degenerative changes had occurred in the cervical spine with production of bony ridges in the anterior wall of the shortened canal and marked bulging of the ligamenta flava. The dural sac was indented over the bony bars anteriorly (Fig. 2.9) and was abnormally thickened and adherent to the posterior longitudinal ligament. The sac was folded "like a concertina" (Breig, 1960) posteriorly (Fig. 2.10) and there were tough

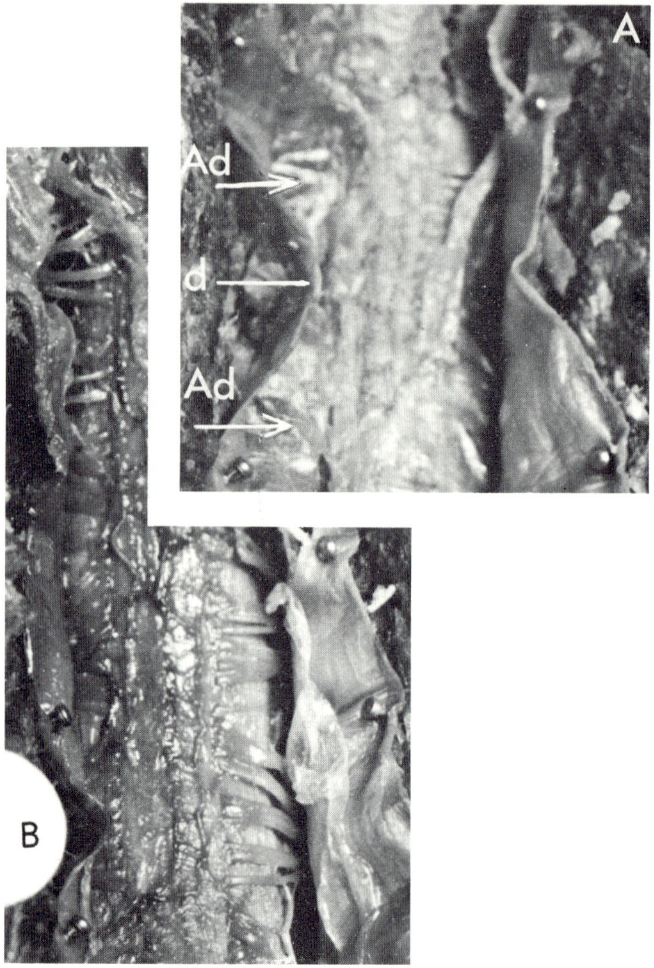

Fig. 2.11A and B (Posterior view of same case as Figs. 9 and 10).

A. The dura has been opened, note that it is tethered at (d) by adhesions (Ad). The arachnoid was unusually thick, opaque and stringy in texture.

B. The arachnoid mater has been opened up. Note the free dorsal rootlets on the right, and the fixed ones on the left at C5 and C6, rootlets above these are free

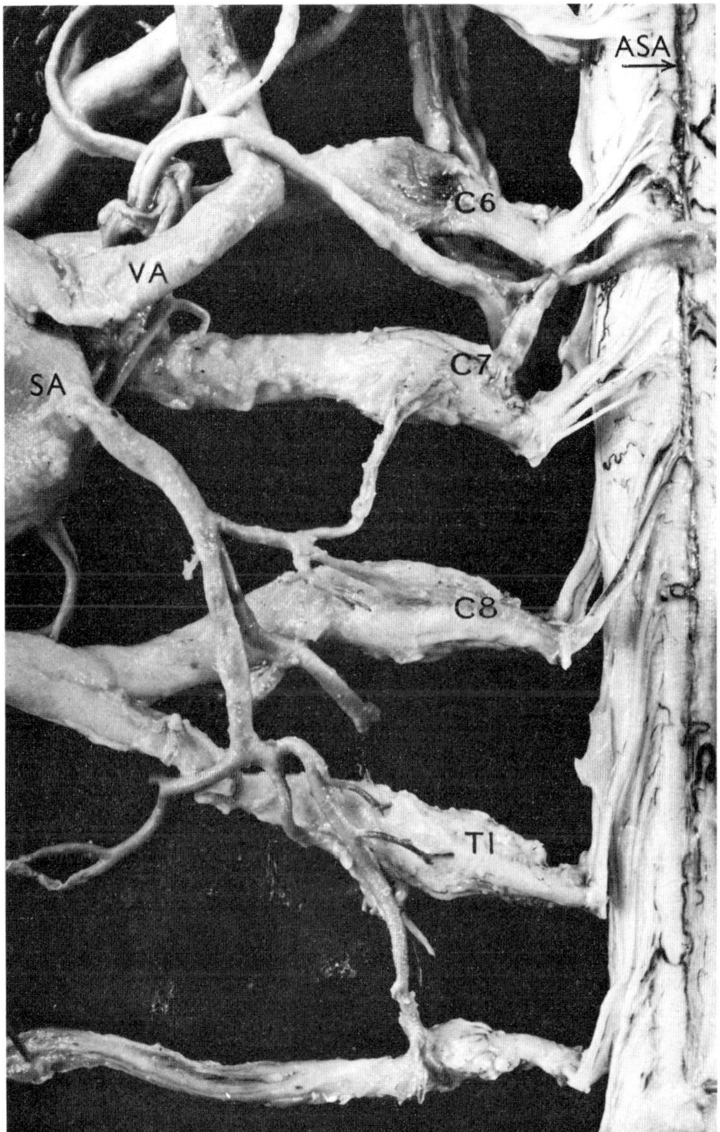

Fig. 2.12 Fixed right brachial plexus from case 10, aged 78 years (Abdullah) showing gross kinking of nerve roots due to shortening of the spinal canal following degeneration of intervertebral discs.

A.S.A. = anterior spinal artery
S.A. = subclavian artery
V.A. = vertebral artery

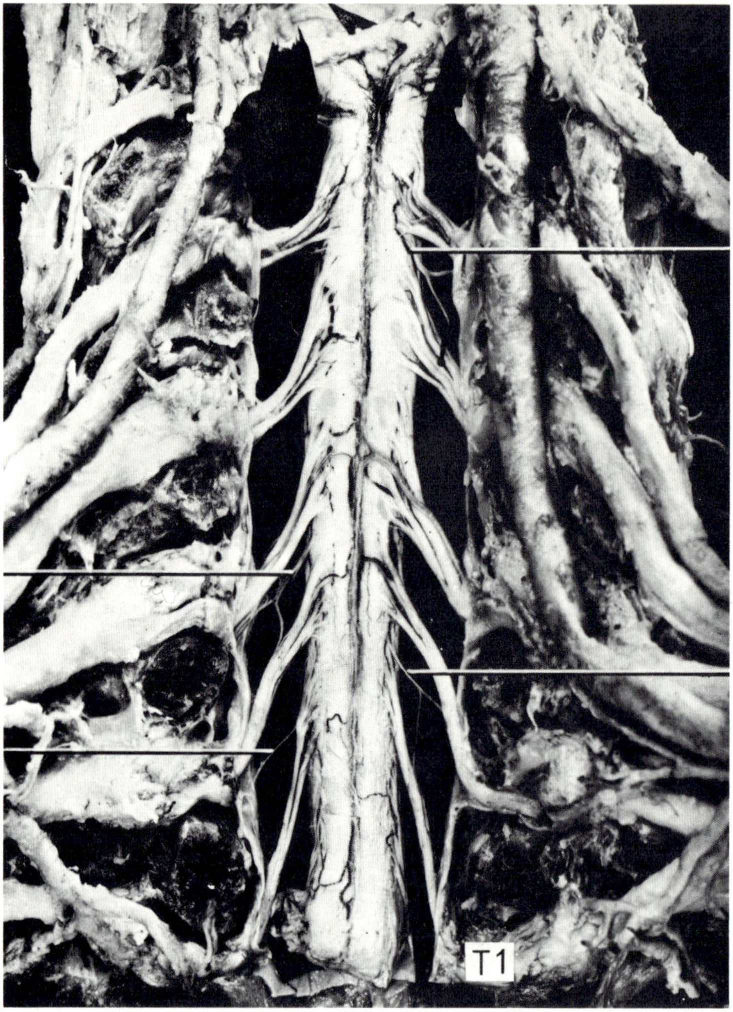

Fig. 2.13 Case 12 (Abdullah) anterior view of roots of brachial plexus showing four rootlets which each contribute to two segmental nerves

adhesions between the dura and arachnoid (Fig. 2.11a) and others within the subarachnoid space (Fig. 2.11b).

Since these acquired abnormalities of the cervical spine affect the related nervous and vascular structures, it follows that any congenital abnormality of the atlanto-occipital region and cervical vertebrae which causes abnormal restriction of movement or alignment of the bones is also likely to disturb neuro-osseous and neurovascular relations.

The roots of cervical nerves are not only at risk within the spinal canal and at the intervertebral foramina, but also after they emerge. The nerves rest on shelves formed by the true transverse and costal elements of the transverse processes (Figs. 2.1 and 2.2). From above downwards these shelves slope at different angles, and whilst resting on them, the nerves may give attachment to some of the fibres of the scalene muscles which elevate and suspend the first ribs and contract continuously and rhythmically at each inspiratory phase. Grossly tortuous vertebral vessels may also distort the nerves and lower cervical ganglia which are trapped between them and the transverse processes (Abdullah, 1958; Abdullah and Bowden, 1960).

THE LOCALISATION OF NEUROLOGICAL LESIONS ASSOCIATED WITH CERVICAL SPONDYLOSIS

It is well recognised that the level of the most severe bony changes does not necessarily correspond with the segmental level of neurological damage. There are two reasons for this, the first is due to the disproportionate growth of the cord and canal. The 1st thoracic segment of the cord lies opposite the 7th cervical vertebra, and the upper rootlets of the lower cervical and 1st thoracic nerves cross two intervertebral discs and normally the lower rootlets of these two nerves only cross one disc. The second reason is that severe degeneration of the discs may shorten the vertebral canal to such an extent that the spinal cord which is unaltered in length, drops down relative to the bones. The spinal nerve roots may then become acutely folded as they travel towards the intervertebral foramina and since the effect is cumulative, the lowest roots are the most severely affected (Fig. 2.12).

Localisation of the neurological segments requires knowledge of the distribution of sensory, motor and autonomic components in segmental nerves. There is no clear cut demarcation between the segments of the cord, a single dorsal or ventral rootlet may divide and contribute to two spinal nerves (Fig. 2.13) and the origin and form of the brachial plexus is not invariably the same (p. 33). Despite these variants a lesion may be localised with reasonable accuracy, if the picture of sensory, motor and autonomic function is assessed as a whole.

The Segmental Distribution of Sensory Fibres

There is still some uncertainty about the precise arrangement of segmental sensory innervation of skin, as will be seen by comparing Fig. 14a and b and Fig. 15a and b based on the work of Head and Foerster and of Keegan and Garrett (1948). For practical purposes the similarities are more important than the dissimilarities. Both schemes indicate that the lower fibres of the cervical plexus supply the cap of the shoulder, the fifth and sixth cervical roots supply the lateral side of the arm and forearm; the hand is innervated by the 6th, 7th and 8th nerves; and the latter extends into

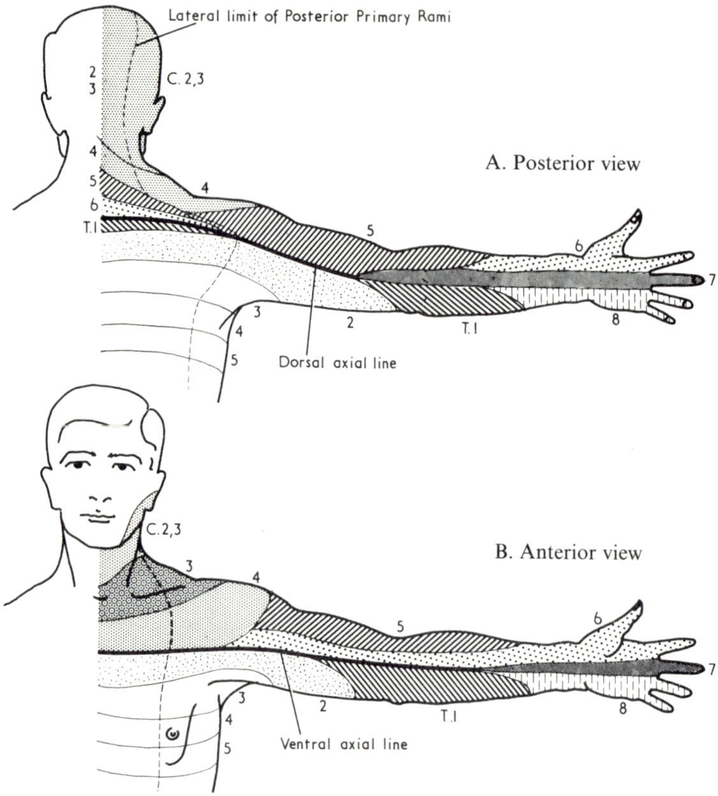

Fig. 2.14A and B Segmental innervation of skin according to Head and Foerster

the forearm. The first thoracic segment innervates the medial side of the arm and forearm. Some inconsistencies would be expected from the anatomical variations already indicated above.

The picture is more confused in relation to the segmental sensory supply of skeletal and articular structures. Inman and Saunders (1944) found no correspondence between the dermatomes and segmental distribution to underlying deep structures. Various stimuli evoked dull, aching or boring, diffuse pain which radiated and was sometimes associated with vasomotor disturbances such as sweating, blanching and nausea. Visceral pain is referred in some cases to well defined segmental areas, e.g. pain over the point of the shoulder (C3, C4) may be associated with acute cholecystitis and other causes of diaphragmatic irritation.

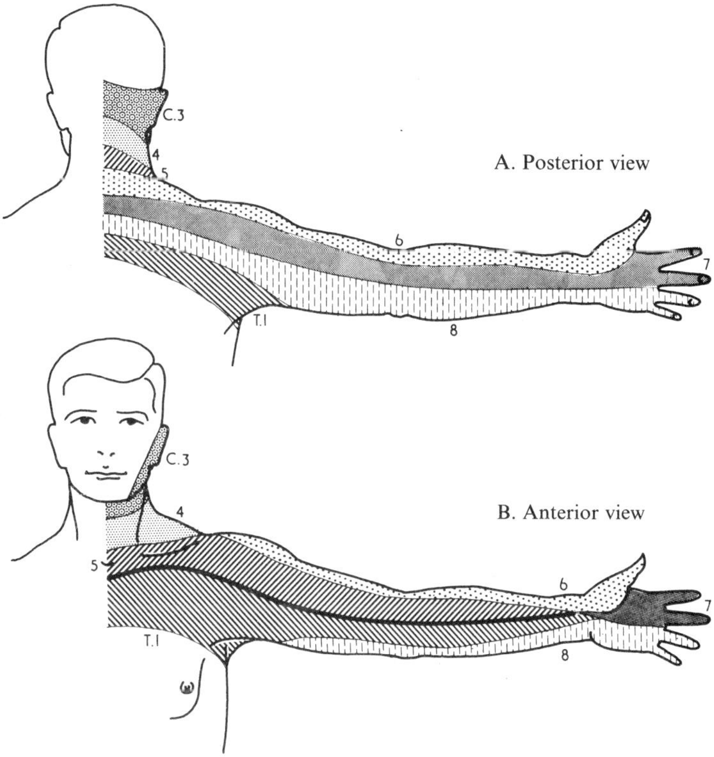

Fig. 2.15A and B Segmental innervation of skin according to Keegan and Garrett

Motor fibres

The segmental supply of individual muscles is given in larger standard textbooks of anatomy and neurology, but useful information is gained by attempting to elicit reflex contractions of biceps brachii and brachioradialis (C5, C6) and of triceps (C7, C8). The intrinsic muscles of the hand are innervated by the first thoracic segment, but this is not invariably the sole source of supply, the 8th cervical and sometimes the 7th segment may also be involved.

Autonomic fibres

Preganglionic sympathetic fibres are derived from the lateral horn of grey matter of the thoracic and upper two lumbar segments of the spinal cord. Occasionally the upper limit extends into the 8th cervical segment, but the fibres emerge only in the anterior roots of the thoracic and upper two or three lumbar nerves. The ouflow from T1 and T2 is destined for the superior cervical ganglion and the post ganglionic fibres supply the head and neck. If these pre-ganglionic fibres are damaged, there will be loss of sweating on the affected side of the face; ptosis, meiosis and enophtholmos, i.e. Horner's syndrome, and occasionally there is perceptible flattening of the nostril on the same side. When this syndrome is associated with paralysis of intrinsic muscles of the hand after an acute injury, the prognosis is extremely poor because it indicates a lesion close to the cord. If the root has been avulsed, a myelogram shows a leak through a tear in the dura. Regeneration of the nerve is impossible and definitive treatment can be arranged without undue delay. It may involve an amputation.

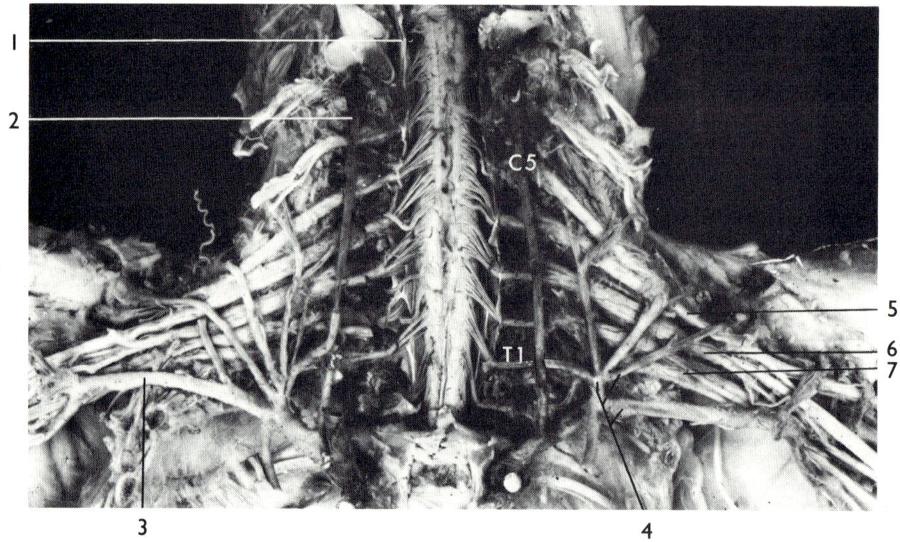

Fig. 2.16 Foetus, 16 weeks (Abdullah). Classical arrangement of symmetrical brachial plexuses dissected to show the origin and course of constituent nerves, and the relations of vessels and meninges. 1 Cut edge of dura mater; 2 Vertebral artery; 3 Subclavian artery; 4 Subclavian artery and branches supplying the plexus and surrounding tissues; 5, 6, 7 Upper, middle and lower trunks of the brachial plexus

The outflow of pre-ganglionic fibres for the upper limb is not necessarily symmetrical, but it may extend from about the 2nd to the 10th thoracic segments.

There are three sympathetic ganglia in the cervical chain. Pre-ganglionic fibres for the head and upper four cervical segments end in the superior ganglion, post ganglionic fibres travel to the head on the walls of blood vessels; those for spinal nerves leave the ganglion in gray rami which connect with each spinal nerve. The 5th and 6th roots receive fibres from the middle ganglion and the 7th and 8th from the inferior one. When the latter is linked with the 1st thoracic, they form the stellate ganglion. The heart also receives fibres from the cervical sympathetic chain. Sympathetic disturbances in the distribution of spinal nerves are demonstrated by alterations in sweating and in vaso-motor responses. Sympathetic fibres also innervate the *arrectores pili* in hairy skin.

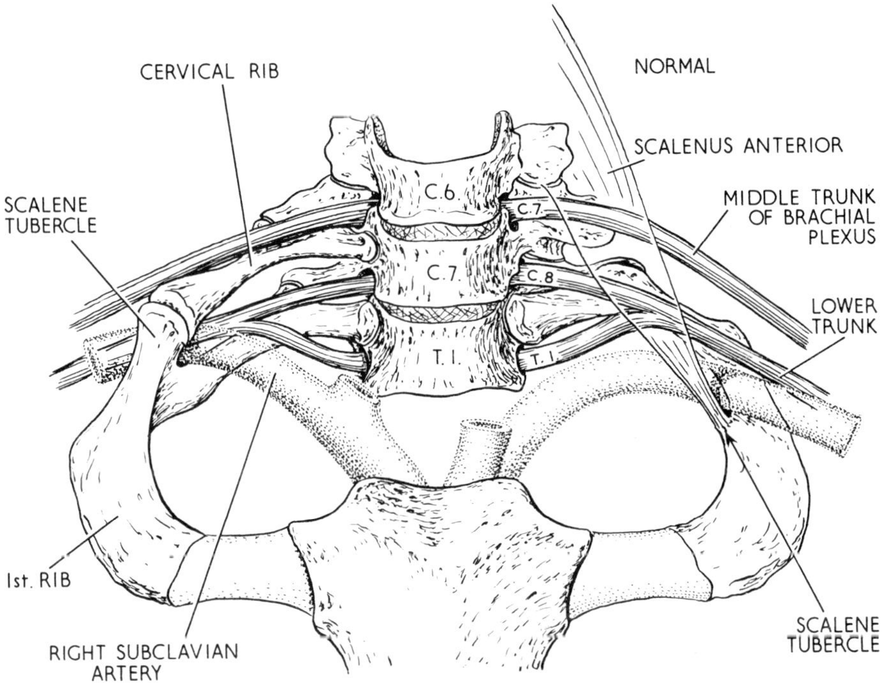

Fig. 2.17 Drawing of a dissecting room specimen of a right cervical rib, no history was available

The Brachial Plexus

The roots of the brachial plexus emerge between scalenus anterior and medius to form the upper, middle and lower trunks. The typical arrangement is shown in Fig. 2.16. The upper roots travel down with varying and decreasing degrees of obliquity and the contribution from first thoracic nerve travels upwards from below the neck of the first rib to cross its flat upper surface either deep to, or just behind, the subclavian artery. The trunks converge and divide into anterior and posterior secondary divisions behind the middle third of the clavicle at the inlet of the axilla. These divisions form the lateral, medial and posterior cords which gradually spiral round the subclavian artery in a clockwise direction on the right side and anticlockwise on the left. They come to lie in relation to the artery in the positions indicated by their names. In their passage from the spinal canal to the axilla the nerve roots and their derivatives change direction several times and they are moved with movements of the shoulder. A drop in the shoulder girdle, most commonly occurring in middle aged women, increases tension in the neurovascular bundle. A tendinous or true bony cervical rib ties the lowest roots and lower trunk down on to the first rib and thus restricts freedom of

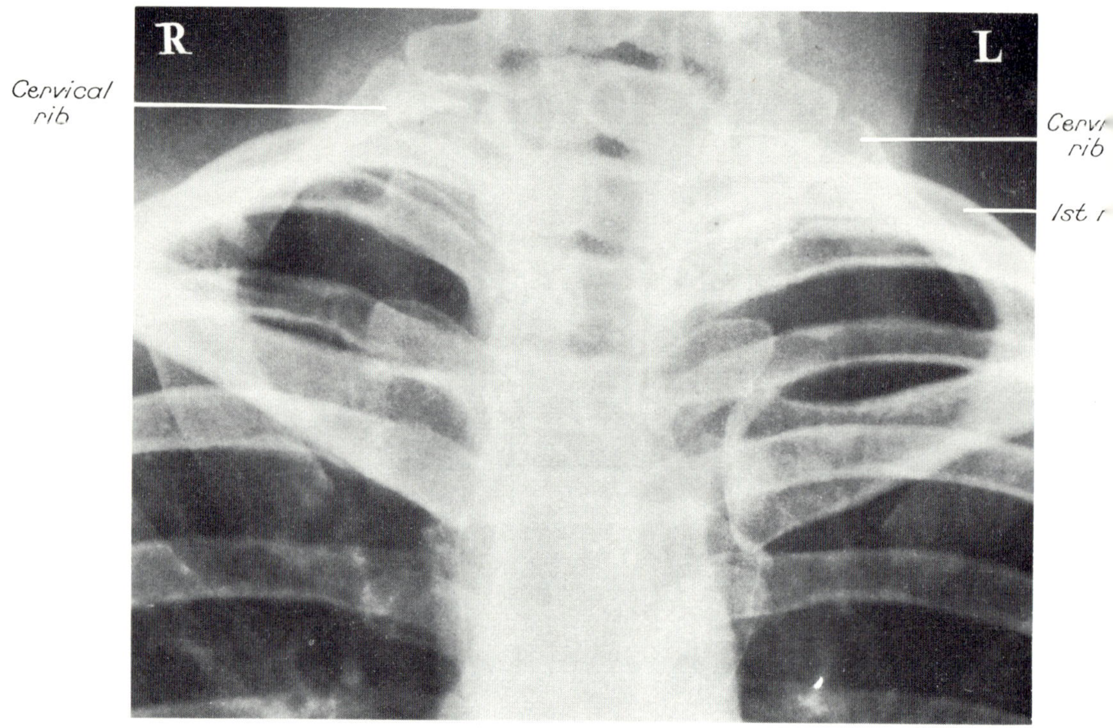

Fig. 2.18 Bilateral cervical ribs. The patient, a woman of 42 years, complained of pain and tingling for four months over the inner side of the *right* hand and ring and little fingers. No objective sensory loss could be detected on clinical examination, but the hypothenar muscles were weak. There were no signs of vascular disturbance (Thanks are due to Mr. Carmo Trindade for the X-ray plate and permission to publish the clinical data)

movement. This may lead to signs and symptoms of an irritative or paralytic lesion of the 8th cervical or 1st thoracic nerves. In some instances there may be circulatory disturbances due to spasm, stenosis or thrombosis of the subclavian artery.

The formation and arrangement of the brachial plexus are not constant. The plexus may be pre- or post-fixed, and the 7th nerve may contribute to the inner cord as well as to the lateral and posterior ones. The left and right plexuses in an individual are not always symmetrical (Bowden, Abdullah and Gooding, 1967). For these and other reasons indicated earlier (p. 27) exact localisation of the level of neurological damage and correlation between this and the damage in bones and joints may prove difficult without meticulous clinical examination coupled with radiology and possibly electromyography and measurement of nerve conduction times.

Much still remains unknown, and one of the most important problems is the mechanism by which irreparable ischaemic damage is produced. Gross distortion of root sleeves and angulation of nerves is not necessarily associated with neurological damage. Possibly the rate at which these encroachments occur may be one of the important factors. If the changes are slow, the tissues may stretch slowly and accommodate gradually to their surroundings.

It is exceedingly difficult to devascularise the spinal cord in an experimental animal in which the vessels resemble those of man (Gooding, 1964). Thromboses in spinal vessels have rarely been found in postmortems of patients who have become paraplegic after relatively trivial acute trauma, or insidious, but progressive damage to the spinal column. Nevertheless the necrotic changes in the cord are clearly in the distribution of either the anterior or posterior spinal arteries (Brain, Northfield and Wilkinson, 1952; Trevor Hughes, 1966). A prolonged spasm of the vessels has been suggested by Davies, Solomon and Levene (1958). Lastly, in the face of evidence of irreversible and often progressive anatomical and functional changes in the cervical column and its related joints it is difficult to explain the transience of neurological signs and symptoms found in many cases.

Acknowledgments

Grateful thanks are due to my colleagues Dr. Sajidah Abdullah and to Mr. Michael Gooding; to Mrs. Audrey Besterman for the drawings; the Photographic Department of the Royal Free Hospital School of Medicine and in particular to Miss Frances Ellis and Mrs. P. Thomas, and to Mr. Carmo Trindade for the radiograph of the cervical ribs, and to him and Dr. Duncan G. Troup for helpful discussions.

References

Abdullah, S. (1958), "Studies of the anatomy of the human brachial plexus with special reference to its blood supply", Thesis for M.Sc. University of London.

Abdullah, S. and Bowden, R. E. M. (1960), *Proc. roy. Soc. Med.*, **53**, 203.

Bakke, S. N. (1931), *Acta radiol., Stockh.*, suppl. 13.

Beadle, O. A. (1931), "The intervertebral disc", *Spec. Rep. Ser. med. Res. Coun.*, H.M.S.O. Lond., No. 161.

Biemond, A. (1951), *Brain,* **74**, 300.

Bowden, R. E. M., Abdullah, S. and Gooding, M. R. (1967), " Anatomy of the cervical spine, membranes, spinal cord, nerve roots and brachial plexus. 10–97 ", in *Cervical Spondylosis and other disorders of the cervical spine*, ed. Lord Brain and Marcia Wilkinson, Wm. Heinemann Medical Books Ltd., London.

Brain, W. R., Northfield, D. W. C. and Wilkinson, M. (1952), *Brain*, **75**, 187.

Breig, A. (1960), *Biomechanics of the central nervous system,* Almqvist and Wiksells, Stockholm.

Brewerton, (1966), *Brit. med. J.*, **i**, 253.

Bull, J. W. D. (1951), *Modern Trends in Neurology*, ed. A. Feiling, Butterworth and Co., London, 600 pp.

Coventry, M. B., Ghormley, R. K. and Kernohan, J. W. (1945a), *J. Bone Jt. Surg.*, **27**, 105.

Coventry, M. B., Ghormley, R. K. and Kernohan, J. W. (1945b), *J. Bone Jt. Surg.*, **27**, 233.

Coventry, M. B., Ghormley, R. K. and Kernohan, J. W. (1945c), *J. Bone Jt. Surg.*, **27**, 460.

Davies, A., Solomon, B. and Levene, A. (1958), *Brit. med. J.*, **2**, 654.

Davis, P. R. (1960), *Actes VIe Cong. Int. sc. Antrop. Ethnol.*, 443.

Davis, P. R. (1966), personal communication.

Davis, P. R. and Rowland, H. A. K. (1965), *J. Bone Jt. Surg.*, **47B**, 61.

Fielding, J. W. (1957), *J. Bone Jt. Surg.*, **39A**, 1280.

Frykholm, R. (1951a), *Acta chir. scand.*, **101**, 345.

Frykholm, R. (1951b), *Acta chir. scand.*, **102**, 10.

Frykholm, R. (1951c), *Acta chir. scand.*, **102**, 93.

Frykholm, R. (1951d), *Acta chir. scand.*, suppl. **160**.

Gooding, M. R. (1964), *A study of some aspects of the blood supply of the spinal cord.* Thesis for M.Sc. University of London.

Hughes, J. Trevor (1966), *Pathology of the Spinal Cord*, Lloyd-Luke, London.

Hutchinson, E. C. and Yates, P. O. (1956), *Brain*, **79**, 319.

Inman, V. T. and Saunders, J. B. de C. M. (1944). *J. Nerv. and Ment. Dis.*, **99**, 660.

Keegan, J. J. and Garrett, F. D. (1948), *Anat. Rec.*, **102**, 409.

McRae, D. L. (1960). *Amer. J. Roentgenol.*, **84**, 3.

Mixter, W. J. (1951), *Modern Trends in Neurology*, ed. Feiling, Butterworth and Co., London, 511 pp.

O'Connell, J. E. A. (1955), *Brit. J. Surg.*, **43**, 225.

Penning, L. (1961), *J. belge Radiol.*, **44**, 551.

Penning, L. (1968), *Functional Pathology of the Cervical Spine*, Excerpta Medica Foundation, Amsterdam, New York, London, Paris, Milan, Tokyo, Buenos Aires.

Penning, L. and van der Zwaag, P. (1966), *Acta radiol.*, **5**, 1090.

Puky, P. de (1935), *Acta orthopaed. scand.*, **6**, 338.

Stoltmann, H. F. and Blackwood, W. (1964), *Brain*, **87**, 45.

Todd, T. W. and Pyle, S. I. (1928), *Amer. J. phys. Anthrop.*, **12**, 321.

Werne, S. (1957), *Acta orthopaed. scand.*, suppl. **23**.

Zeitler, E. and Markuske, H. (1962), *Fortschr. Röntgenstr.*, **96**, 87.

Chapter III

Pathology

MARCIA WILKINSON

In cervical spondylosis the degenerative changes in the intervertebral discs lead to secondary changes in the adjacent vertebrae. The changes in the cervical spine may affect one or more nerve roots, the cervical cord at one or more levels or may cause simultaneous damage to the nerve roots and cord.

Pathogenesis

Many writers have shown that radiological changes in the cervical spine are not necessarily associated with the production of symptoms. Whether or not symptoms do result depend on several factors. Some of these factors are mechanical and include the sagittal diameter of the spinal canal, the size and attachments of the dentate ligament, the presence of root-sleeve fibrosis and of intradural adhesions. Vascular factors may also play a part because the main blood supply of the cervical cord usually comes from two or three radicular arteries and these may be involved by the spondylotic process. Compression of the cord when it occurs is often incomplete or intermittent. It is probable that in any individual patient more than one factor is operating.

The intervertebral discs

The intervertebral discs lie between the bodies of the vertebrae and their thickness varies in different regions of the column and in different parts of the same disc. They are thicker in front than behind in the cervical region and thus contribute to the anterior convexity of this part of the column. Changes in the normal structure of the disc in patients with cervical spondylosis is one of the main causes of the alteration of the normal curve of the cervical spine. The discs are adherent by their surfaces to the layers of hyaline cartilage which cover the upper and under surface of the bodies of the vertebrae and they are also continuous with the anterior and posterior ligaments.

The disc itself is composed of two parts. The periphery is denser than the centre and has its fibres arranged in concentric lamellae. In the vertical plane the fibres are arranged obliquely and angulated in opposite directions in successive lamellae. These peripheral lamellae combine to form that part of the disc known as the annulus fibrosus. The inner part of the disc, the nucleus pulposus, is composed of a fine fibrous matrix containing angular cells which form a reticular structure, and is a soft pulpy highly elastic substance which in young people is under positive pressure. Petter (1933) found that there was a very definite expansion in the lumbar intervertebral disc upon its removal from the body and there was a further expansion when the annulus fibrosus was sectioned, the total being 1·08 mm. The average pressure required to reduce this expansion was 32 lb per square inch. Rupture of the anterior or posterior spinal ligaments allow protrusion of the nucleus pulposus and, in addition to the internal pressure of 32 lb per square inch, the pressure on the disc on standing may rise to 100 lb per square inch or exceptionally on straining to 300 lb per square inch.

The intervertebral discs constitute about one-fourth of the length of the vertebral column in the cervical region. Bull (1948) estimated that the nucleus pulposus constituted about 15 per cent of the volume of a disc and that in the cervical region the maximum volume of the nucleus pulposus which could be extruded would, if spherical,

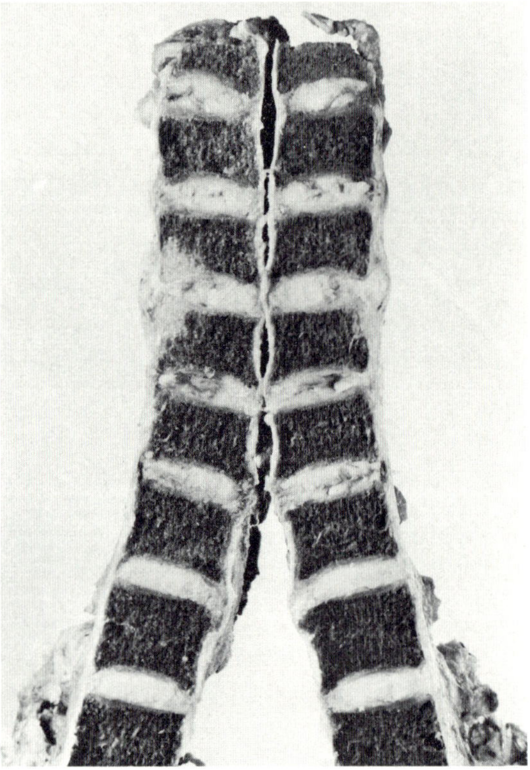

Fig. 3.1 Sagittal section of the cervical spine showing degeneration of the intervertebral discs and protrusion of the C4–5 disc with some sclerosis of adjacent parts of vertebral bodies

have a diameter of 0·7 cm. From this it is clear that seldom, if ever, is the protrusion of the nucleus pulposus alone sufficient to cause compression of the spinal cord although a lateral protrusion may easily compress the appropriate nerve root. This is borne out by the fact that traumatic lesions in young people usually cause a root lesion and that cord compression occurs only if there is a fracture-dislocation. In older people the picture is more complicated because in addition to the protrusion of the nucleus pulposus there is often osteophyte formation with or without root-sleeve fibrosis (Frykholm, 1951).

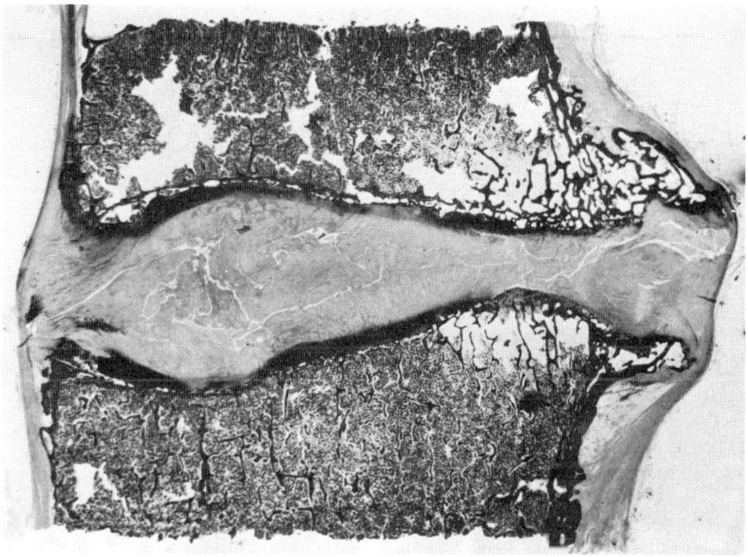

Fig. 3.2 Sagittal section of cervical spine through transverse bar at C4–5 showing disc protrusion and changes in the adjacent vertebrae

Püschel (1930) found that the water content of the disc is highest in the newborn and that it decreased with age. He also found that it was higher in the nucleus pulposus than in the annulus fibrosus. The ratio of the water content of the annulus to that of the nucleus remains approximately the same until the fifth decade, when rapid loss occurs in the nucleus pulposus and this is accompanied by degenerative changes. This is of considerable clinical interest as most patients first complain of symptoms after the age of 50. Saunders and Inman (1939) observed a close correlation between the elasticity and water content of the nucleus pulposus. They considered that progressive desiccation was a major factor in the destruction of the disc and that such a disc was much more susceptible to trauma than a normal one.

In cervical spondylosis osteophytes may occur at any point on the margins of the vertebral bodies (Figs. 3.1 and 3.2). The formation of osteophytes is probably secondary to degenerative and/or traumatic lesions of the intervertebral discs and of the articular cartilages of the vertebral bodies (Fig. 3.3). The osteophytes project outwards from the margins of the vertebral bodies and cracks and erosions may be present in the articular cartilages (Fig. 3.4). Desiccation and other changes in the nuclei pul-

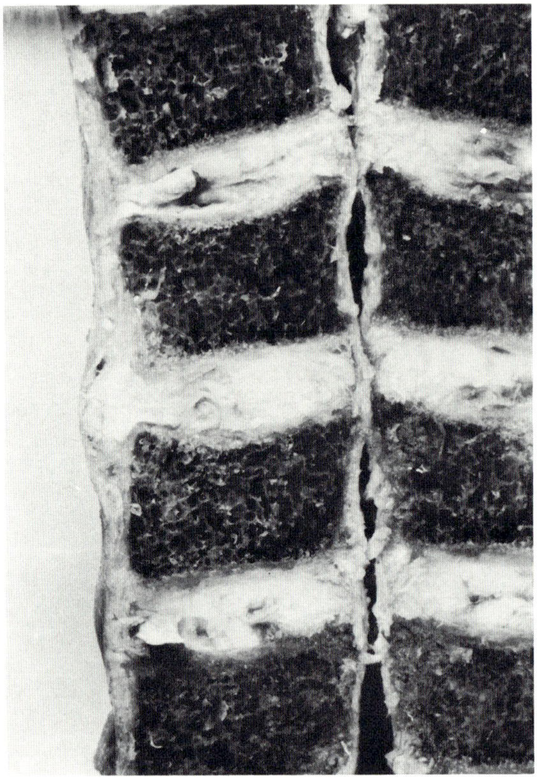

Fig. 3.3 Sagittal section of cervical spine showing disc protrusion and fissuring and degenerative changes in the discs

posi take place with bulging and sometimes rupture of the annulus fibrosus. If the protrusion formed by the osteophytes and ruptured disc projects posteriorly or posterolaterally from the vertebral body this protrusion may encroach upon either the spinal canal or intervertebral foramen and thus become a potential cause of pressure on the cervical cord and/or the cervical nerve roots.

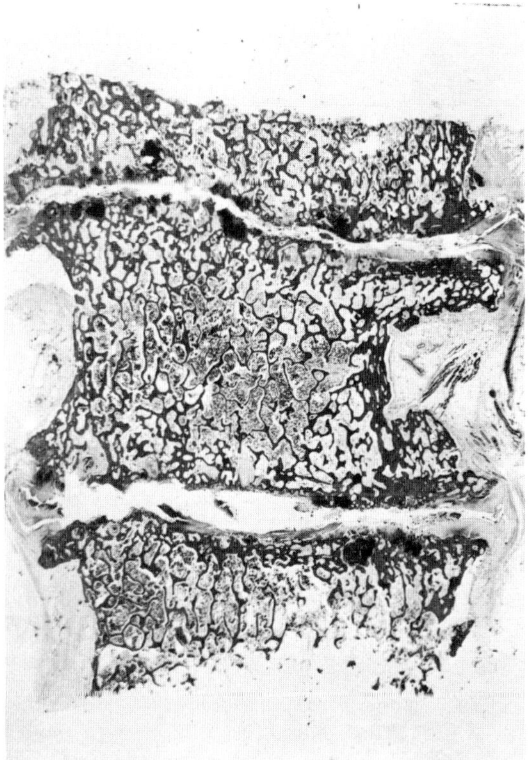

Fig. 3.4 Sagittal section of cervical spine showing disc degeneration and protrusion. Note the almost complete obliteration of disc space and the extensive associated bony changes

The spinal canal

The actual size of the cervical spinal canal is very important because where there is a big canal the likelihood of cord compression is very much reduced. The average sagittal diameter of the cervical spinal canal is 17 mm and in the cervical region the average antero-posterior diameter of the cord is 10 mm. Therefore in the average individual there is unlikely to be cord compression unless there are gross changes in the cervical spine. If, however, the diameter of the canal is less than average a much smaller protrusion will cause cord compression as the antero-posterior diameter of the cord varies only slightly. Wolf, Khilnani and Malis (1956) measured the antero-posterior diameter of the spinal canal in 200 normal adults and found that from C3–7 the average measurement was 17 mm and this was confirmed by Burrows (1963). The sagittal diameter is greatest at the foramen magnum where it is 22·9 mm and is least at the 4th cervical vertebra where the average measurement is 17·7 mm. Burrows also measured the sagittal diameter of the spinal cord in the cervical region using autotomography during lumbar air encephalography and confirmed the findings of Lowman and Finkelstein (1942) that the cord measured 10 mm in a sagittal direction at C1 and was only slightly narrower at C7. Payne and Spillane (1957) measured the sagittal diameter of the cervical spinal canal in patients with myelopathy due to cervical spondylosis and found that in these patients the average measurement of the canal was 14 mm

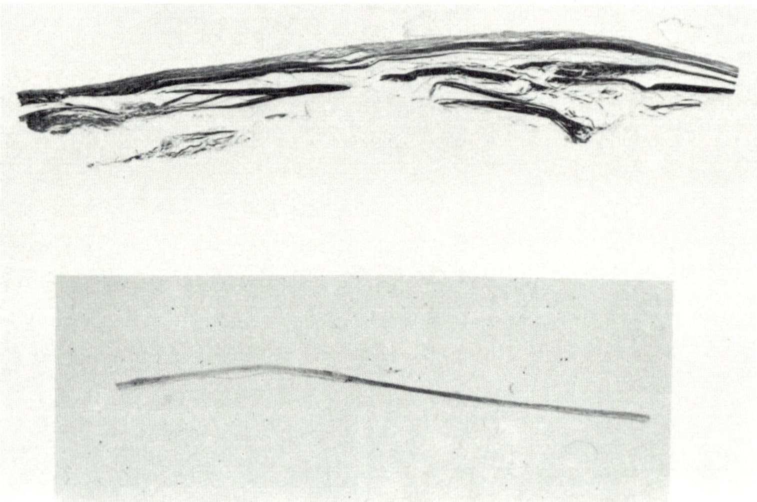

Fig. 3.5 Section of cervical dura mater C2–4 in cervical spondylosis (top) compared with dura mater from the dorsal region of the same patient

—that is to say about 3 mm less than the average. Since the actual amount of degenerative change present is likely to be the same in a patient with a wide canal as in a patient with a narrow canal, the diminished sagittal diameter of the canal is of considerable significance in cervical spondylosis. The bony limits of the sagittal diameter can be measured (Chapter V, p. 84) and it must be remembered that the actual diameter of the canal may be less than it appears radiologically because not all the tissues which reduce the size of the canal cast a radiographic shadow. That is to say the measurement of the distance between the spur on the inferior posterior aspect of the vertebral body and the base of the spinous process of the vertebra below is the maximum possible size of the canal at that point. In practice if this measurement is 11 mm or less, cord compression is likely to occur.

The most common causes of reduction of the sagittal diameter are posterior osteophytes and infolding of the ligamenta flava. Wilkinson (1960) showed that the posterior osteophytes might reduce the sagittal diameter by up to 3 mm and Love and Walsh (1940) demonstrated that thickening of the ligamenta flava might also act as a posterior compressing agent. Taylor (1951) found that in hyperextension of the cervical spine there was marked encroachment upon the mid-cervical cord opposite the interspaces due to infolding of the ligamenta flava and this finding was confirmed by Payne and Spillane, and by Stoltman and Blackwood (1964). In some cases the cervical cord may be compressed from in front by posterior osteophytes and from behind by the ligamenta flava. In these patients there will be signs of posterior column compression in addition to the signs of cortico-spinal tract involvement.

If adhesions are present a myelopathy is more likely to occur. Adhesions are often found at operation in patients with cervical spondylosis. These lie between the dura and the arachnoid, as well as between the arachnoid and the pia, and are probably due to a chronic degenerative process rather than to an infective one. Similar changes are always found if the patient has had a previous cervical laminectomy. The myelogram in these patients shows ragged diffuse areas of poor filling. After laminectomy the dura may be thickened and adherent to the posterior longitudinal ligament (Brain, Northfield and Wilkinson, 1952) (Fig. 3.5).

The dentate ligament anchors the dura to the lateral wall of the spinal canal. In some patients this ligament is a delicate filamentous thread but in others it is a coarse fibrous band. Kahn (1947) suggested that tethering of the cord by the dentate ligament was important and Bedford, Bosanquet and Russell (1952) found that there were areas of cord degeneration related to the thickened dentate ligaments.

Congenital abnormalities of the cervical spine

Many different types of congenital abnormality of the cervical spine may be found (see Chapter V) but the most common abnormality is fusion of two or more cervical vertebrae (the Klippel-Feil abnormality). Fusion may occur between any two vertebrae but symptoms are most likely to occur if the fusion is between C4–5, C5–6 or C6–7. Maximum movement occurs above or below the fused vertebrae and spondylotic changes tend to occur at those levels and this is probably associated with the extra movement which occurs. These spondylotic changes will diminish the effective sagittal diameter of the spinal canal. In other types of congenital abnormality of the cervical spine there may also be narrowing of the spinal canal and if there are associated spondylotic changes these again will tend to cause spinal cord compression (Fig. 3.6).

The zygapophyseal joints

The zygapophyseal or interpedicular joints are synovial joints formed by the articulation of the adjacent superior and inferior facets of the vertebral pedicles. The superior facets are directed upwards, backwards and medially and the inferior downwards, forwards and laterally. The zygapophyseal joints form the posterior and lateral boundaries of the intervertebral foramina.

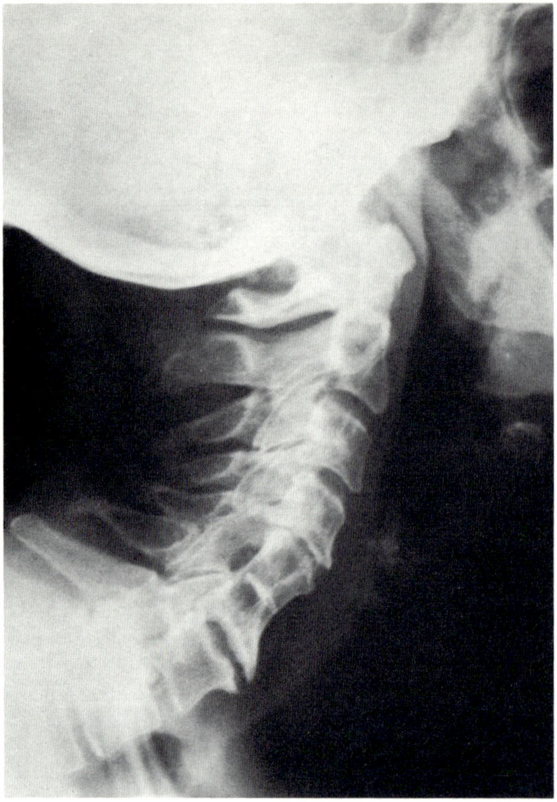

Fig. 3.6 Lateral X-ray of the cervical spine showing fusion of the bodies of the 5th and 6th cervical vertebrae and spondylotic changes at C4–5

Osteoarthritic changes of the zygapophyseal joints are almost as common as changes in the disc. Zygapophyseal changes may occur at levels where the discs are relatively normal and this is most common in the upper cervical regions (C2–3, C3–4). In the lower cervical region where spondylosis is most frequently found osteoarthritis of the zygapophyseal joints is less common. If osteophytes are present on the margins of the articulating facets of the zygapophyseal joints there may be encroachment on the spinal canal and on the intervertebral foramina, mainly from the posterior and lateral aspects. If zygapophyseal joint changes and disc disease are present at the same level the nerve roots are in double jeopardy as the foramen is encroached upon from the posterior and lateral aspect by the changes in the zygapophyseal joints and from the medial aspect by the spondylotic bars. As the cervical vertebral bodies come closer together following disc degeneration, the cervical laminae usually do the same. The upper edge of one cervical lamina may even come to lie inside the lower edge of the lamina above it. This results in shortening and folding of the ligamentum flavum and perhaps degeneration and swelling of this ligament. The enfolded or swollen ligamentum flavum encroaches on the posterior part of the spinal canal and therefore further diminishes the antero-posterior diameter.

Nerve root compression

The spinal nerves are covered by a sheath of dura as they leave the spinal cord, this being known as the dural root pouch. At the bottom of the root pouches there are two openings, the dural root ostia, and each root ostium leads into an individual root-sleeve. The root-sleeves, which are lateral extensions of the dura, are separated by a

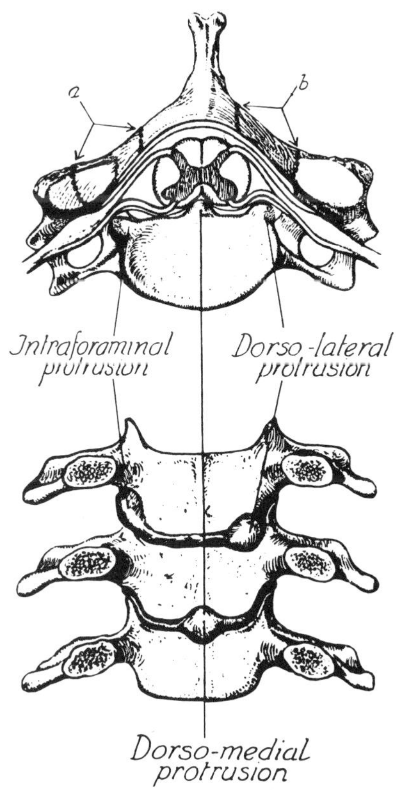

Fig. 3.7 Site of disc protrusions (Frykholm)

small cleft known as the inter-radicular foramen. Between the dural sac and the dorsal root ganglion the two roots lie close together and are called the radicular nerve. Normally this radicular nerve occupies one-fifth to one-fourth of the foramen. Frykholm (1951) has shown that there is a considerable variation in the morphology of the lower cervical nerves and their root pouches, and that, as age advances, they become relatively fixed and, therefore, more liable to damage. He thought that the pathological lesion responsible for radicular symptoms was root-sleeve fibrosis, and that this was characterised by thickening and opacity of the dural root-sleeve and adjacent parts of the dural sac, narrowing or complete abolition of the dural funnel

TABLE 3.1 *Table showing incidence of disc protrusions in patients who came to autopsy*

Patient	*C2–3*	*C3–4*	*C4–5*	*C5–6*	*C6–7*	*C7–T1*	*Total*
1		+	+	+	+		4
2		+	+	+	+		4
3				+	+		2
4				+	+	+	3
5		+					1
6	+	+	+	+	+		5
7		+	+	+			3
8	+	+	+	+	+		5
9	+	+	+	+			4
10	+		+	+	+	+	5
11		+	+	+	+		4
12			+	+			2
13				+			1
14		+	+	+	+		4
15		+		+			2
16		+		+			2
17		+	+	+			3

which forms the root pouch, sharpening of the upper and lower duro-radicular junction which sometimes causes a distinct constriction or notching of the radicular nerve, thickening of the dura at the root ostia, and thickening and fibrosis of the arachnoid membrane in the neighbourhood of the root ostia. Ricard and Masson (1951) suggested that intradural root compression might also be due to the secondary formation of arachnoid cysts.

There are two types of disc lesion which may cause pressure on the radicular nerves or nerve roots (Fig. 3.7). These are a dorso-lateral protrusion which does not invade the intervertebral foramen but may compress the intrameningeal nerve roots against the vertebral laminae, and secondly an intraforaminal protrusion which comes from the uncinate part of the disc and compresses the radicular nerve against the articular process. The extent of root compression is related to the angulation of the radicular nerve and its situation in the foramen, as well as to the size and position of the protrusion. Marginal lipping of the vertebrae and narrowing of the disc lead to secondary osteophyte formation of the articular processes which cause narrowing of the foramen postero-laterally. Wilkinson (1960) found some or all of these changes in 17 patients who came to autopsy (Table 3.1). All had opacity and thickening of the dural root sleeves and adjacent parts of the dural sac of one or more nerve roots and in most there was narrowing of the dural funnel. These patients also showed thickening and fibrosis of the arachnoid in the neighbourhood of the root ostia.

The Blood Supply of the Spinal Cord

There is considerable variation in the pattern of blood vessels in the cervical cord, and the main blood supply usually comes through a few major radicular arteries, the anterior and posterior spinal arteries acting more as connecting links than as a main channel of blood supply. Because the main supply comes through one or more radicular arteries and because these are very liable to be compressed if the degree of cervical spondylosis is marked, the blood supply to the cord is often impaired in patients with cervical spondylosis. This impairment may be either continuous or intermittent and sometimes the maximum impairment only occurs when the head is in a certain position, usually extension. Adamkiewitz (1882) and Kadyi (1889) showed that only one to three radicular arteries contributed to the anterior spinal artery and about three to five lesser branches to the posterior spinal arteries. Herren and Alexander (1939) put the number of radicular contributing arteries to the cervical cord as low as two, while Abdullah (1958) showed that although most spinal roots are accompanied by an artery, their area of blood supply stops in most cases at the root and posterior ganglion and only one or two arteries take part in the spinal cord circulation. Taylor (1964) showed that in a spinal cord injected post-mortem by perfusion of both vertebral arteries at their ante-mortem pressure, only two branches contributing to the anterior spinal artery were seen and in further experiments he showed that if all the radicular arteries are clipped and the vertebral arteries then injected the cord can be supplied only as low as C3–4 from the two anterior spinal branches merging at the foramen magnum. He went on to suggest that on experimental grounds obstruction to the main radicular arteries at the C5–6 level would result in an ischaemic cord lesion extending from C4–T1.

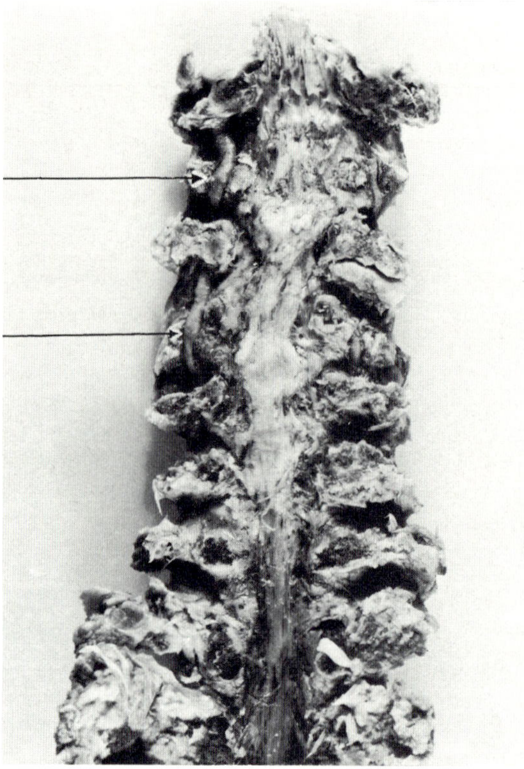

Fig. 3.8 Dissection of posterior aspect of cervical spine showing irregular bosses and bars. The lateral ends of these bars can be seen, arrowed, encroaching on the intervertebral foramina and displacing the vertebral artery posteriorly and laterally

Brain (1956) drew attention to vascular factors in the production of symptoms in a patient with cervical spondylosis. He thought that the earliest changes produced by a protruded disc were circulatory, the veins with their thin walls and low pressure being compressed first, and that, since the flow in them is upwards, an oedema of the anterior or antero-lateral columns would occur at the level of the compression and for some segments below. Similarly, oedema would be produced in the spinal roots compressed.

Arterial blood supply would be affected later, if at all, and either the radicular or anterior spinal arteries might be compressed. Mair and Druckman (1953) noted the correspondence between the areas of demyelination found in the cervical cord and the distribution of the terminal arterioles of the anterior spinal arteries. There were no microscopical changes in the main artery and they suggested that the cause of the demyelination was pressure on the artery by the spondylotic bars. Greenfield (1953) also thought that the anterior spinal artery might be compressed but considered the areas of demyelination were too scattered and circumscribed to be caused by direct pressure. He also mentioned that narrowing of the intervertebral foramina could affect the radicular vessels. Krogdahl and Torgerson (1940) emphasised the likelihood that pressure on the cervical nerves, their contained vessels and the vertebral artery itself, played some part in the causation of myelopathy.

The vertebral arteries

The vertebral arteries may vary considerably in size and one is usually a good deal larger than the other. Hutchinson and Yates (1956), found the left the larger in 51 per cent of cases, the right in 41 per cent and the arteries of equal size in only 8 per cent. The vertebral artery lies within the vertebral canal and on its medial aspect is closely related to the neurocentral joint and passes immediately anterior to the emerging cervical nerve root. Each root is supplied by a small arterial twig. Spondylotic changes of the cervical vertebrae may displace the artery laterally (Fig. 3.8) and in the more severe cases posteriorly also (Pallis, Jones and Spillane, 1954). The degree of displacement depends on the size and position of the bony prominences which arise as a result of spondylotic changes and the displacement of the artery may vary from a gentle curve to a marked distortion. Atheroma of the vertebral artery may also be an important factor in the production of symptoms. Hutchinson and Yates demonstrated that atheroma of this artery within the vertebral canal might cause infarction of the cerebellum. The infarcts result from a critical reduction of blood flow through the vertebral artery in the neck. Where the block is in the cervical part of the vertebral artery the cerebellar infarcts tend to be bilateral, approximately symmetrical and in the territory of the superior cerebellar artery. This block may be complete but it is more often incomplete and obstruction of the blood flow may only occur when the patient turns or extends his head. De Kleyn (1939) showed that rotation and extension of the head to one side obstructed the contralateral vertebral artery while Biemond (1951) found, in a series of patients with arteriosclerosis, that rotation and extension of the head produced nystagmus, dysarthria and a transient abnormality of the plantar responses. Hutchinson and Yates suggested that cervical spondylosis, which is a common condition over the age of 50, and which can distort the vertebral artery, might play a role in obstructing one or other of the vertebral arteries during movements of the cervical spine. Whether or not obstruction occurs depends on the size and extent of the spondylotic boss or bar and its relation to the vertebral artery and/or the main radicular supply artery.

Thrombosis of the anterior spinal artery is a diagnosis which is fairly frequently made but rarely found when a full pathological examination is made. It is probable that more often the symptoms are due to compression of one of the main radicular arteries by osteophytes or adhesions associated with root-sleeve fibrosis, as the anterior spinal artery appears to be more a linking channel than the main source of blood supply to the cord. Hughes and Brownell (1964) described a case in which there was infarction of the anterior part of the spinal cord from C4 down to Th1, and in this case there was thrombosis of the anterior spinal artery and its branches. Severe cervical spondylosis was present and was thought to be the probable cause. In any generalised disorder of the vessels the blood supply of the cervical cord may be impaired and if this is associated with spondylotic changes the liability to an impaired blood supply is increased. Arteriosclerosis, diabetes and syphilis are all conditions in which there may be a generalised impairment of the blood supply and in all these conditions thrombosis of the anterior spinal artery has been reported.

Other vascular changes sometimes observed are apparently aberrant blood vessels coursing between the pia and arachnoid and often associated with an arachnoiditis. It is probable that if there is a degree of vascular insufficiency a significant proportion of the blood supply of the cord may depend on these unusual blood vessels.

Obstruction of the Vertebral Artery

Vertigo, dizziness and weakness of the limbs associated with drop attacks may be due to an insufficient blood supply in the territory of the vertebrobasilar system. These symptoms are often precipitated or exacerbated by movements of the neck and it is probable that if this is the case the intermittent obstruction may be due to compression of the artery by laterally or postero-laterally placed spondylotic bosses or bars. The fact that the vertebral artery could be obstructed either partially or completely by extension and rotation of the head was first demonstrated in the region of the atlas and axis in cadavers by De Kleyn and Nieuwenhuyse (1927) and later by Tatlow and Bammer (1957) and Virtama and Kivalo (1957). Hutchinson and Yates were the first to describe distortion of the vertebral artery by spondylotic outgrowths in cadavers. They described 40 patients in 19 of whom there was an associated atherosclerosis. Later Sheehan, Bauer and Meyer (1960) demonstrated, by means of angiography, distortion of the vertebral artery by the cervical osteophytes and they also showed that extension and rotation of the head increased compression on the side to which the head was rotated. In other patients rotation of the head may cause compression of the vertebral artery as it passes through the transverse process of the atlas on the side away from which the head is rotated.

If there is compression of the vertebral artery by a spondylotic outgrowth decompression may be possible and this has been done in a few patients. In one (Gortvai, 1964), the vertebral artery was found to be severely kinked at the upper margin of the 6th cervical vertebra. A bony spur and a fibro-cartilagenous mass, almost certainly displaced disc material, were removed from the foramen transversarium. Following the removal of this mass the artery appeared to straighten out and pulsate normally, and whereas before the operation this patient was complaining of pain in the neck, weakness of the right limbs, dizziness on standing and attacks of dropping to the ground, following operation he was virtually symptom-free. In this patient's case the situation was made worse by the fact that there was no patent vertebral artery on the opposite side. If there is atheroma of the vertebral artery obstruction of the vessel may be partly intraluminal and, if this is so, external decompression alone may not achieve good results.

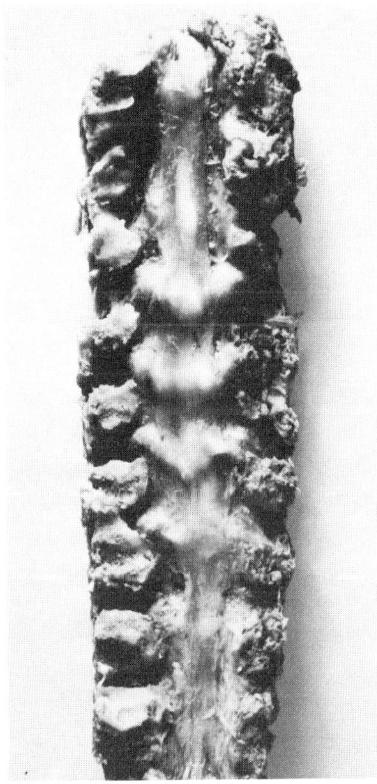

Fig. 3.9 Posterior aspect of bodies of vertebrae showing transverse bosses and bars from the same case as Fig. 3.11

CERVICAL MYELOPATHY

In cervical spondylosis the spinal cord is less frequently involved than the nerve roots but even so spondylotic myelopathy is one of the commonest disorders of the spinal cord during and after middle life and a diagnosis of spondylosis must be considered in any elderly patient who has a spastic paraplegia. The most conspicuous macroscopical features in the spinal canal are the posterior bosses or bars associated with the affected intervertebral discs (Wilkinson, 1960; Hughes, 1966) (Fig. 3.9). The transverse bars may extend across the posterior aspect of the vertebrae or there may be localised bosses either centrally or laterally (Fig. 3.10) or there may be a combination of both. The

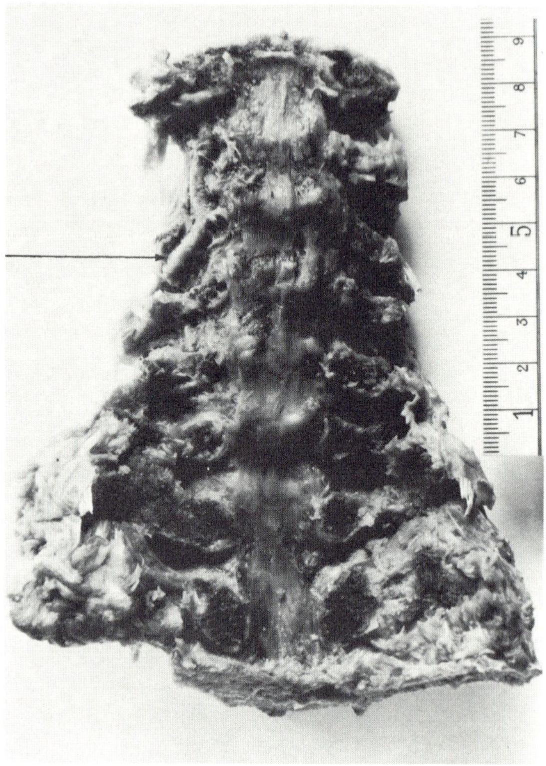

Fig. 3.10 Posterior aspect of bodies of vertebrae showing multiple transverse bars. The left vertebral artery is displaced by the lateral end of the bar corresponding to the disc between C3 and C4 arrowed

lateral end of the bars may encroach on an intervertebral foramina and thereby cause pressure on a nerve root as well as cord compression. Frequently these lesions are found at more than one level. If these bosses or bars are big enough to cause compression, the spinal cord shows indentations corresponding to the spondylotic protrusions

(Figs. 3.11 and 3.12). This appearance may sometimes be exaggerated by post-mortem moulding during fixation, but microscopical examination of the cord in these cases will show localised histological changes. Wilkinson (1960) (Table 3.1) described a series of 17 patients with cervical spondylosis who came to autopsy. Twelve of these had flattening and distortion of the cord, the extent and site of which corresponded to the distribution and size of the bosses and bars on the posterior aspect of the vertebral

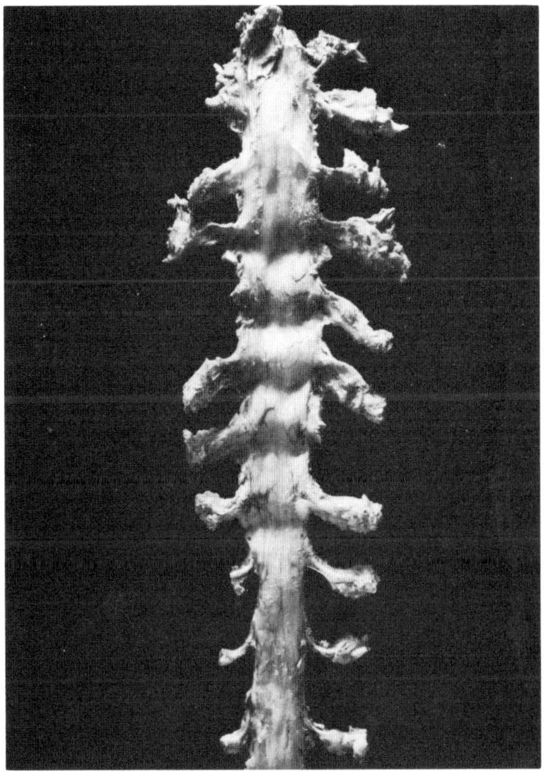

Fig. 3.11 Anterior aspect of cervical cord showing indentations of cord and nerve roots corresponding to the bosses and bars on the posterior aspect of the cervical spine. See Fig. 3.9

column. The main structural change was at C4 in one patient, C5 in four, C6 in two, C7 in two and extended over two or more segments in the other three. In 12 there was demyelination of the lateral column at the site of the lesion (Fig. 3.13). Cephalad to the most damaged segments there was degeneration of the dorsal columns (Fig. 3.14). In the grey matter, nerve-cell damage and loss was sometimes severe (11 patients) and in three there was marked cavitation (Fig. 3.15). Caudad to the lesions there was degeneration in the lateral column. Four of the 17 patients died within 3 weeks of a heavy fall, the main cause of death being compression of the cervical cord at the time of the injury, clearly facilitated by pre-existing cervical spondylosis (Fig. 3.16).

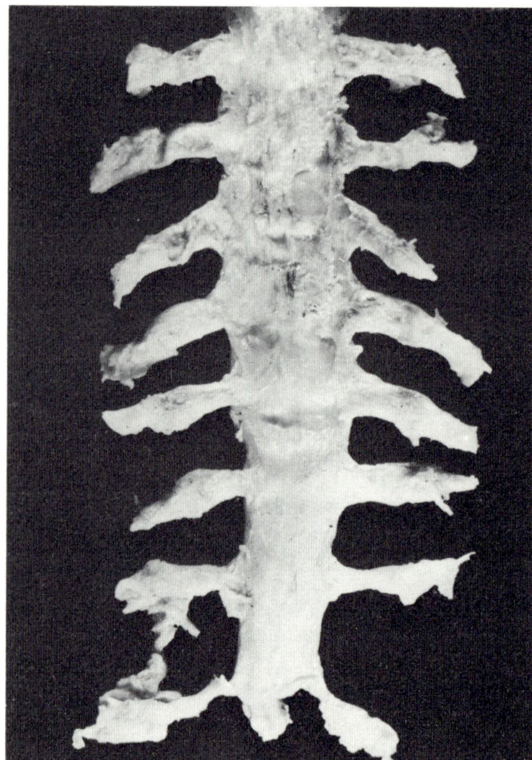

Fig. 3.12 Anterior aspect of cervical cord showing indentations corresponding to the bosses and bars on the posterior aspect of the bodies of the vertebrae. Well-marked root-sleeve fibrosis and dural adhesions are also present

Hughes (1966) considers that in order to justify the pathological diagnosis of myelopathy caused by cervical spondylosis there should be degeneration of the posterior and lateral columns with destruction of grey and white matter. He also points out

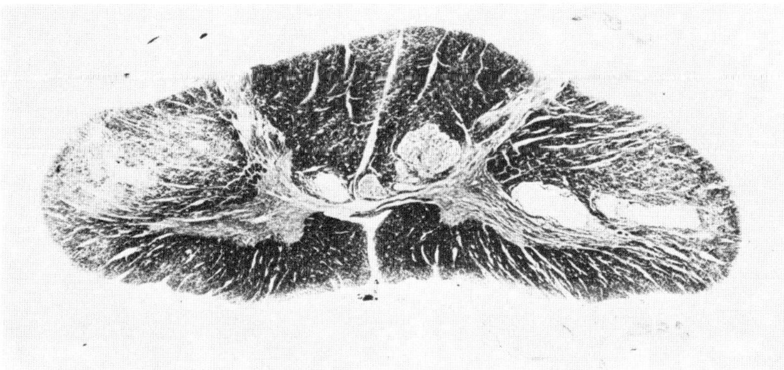

Fig. 3.13 Cervical cord (C4) × 7 showing gross destruction of the cord following injury, most marked in the lateral columns. There is extrusion of necrotic material from lower segments into the posterior column

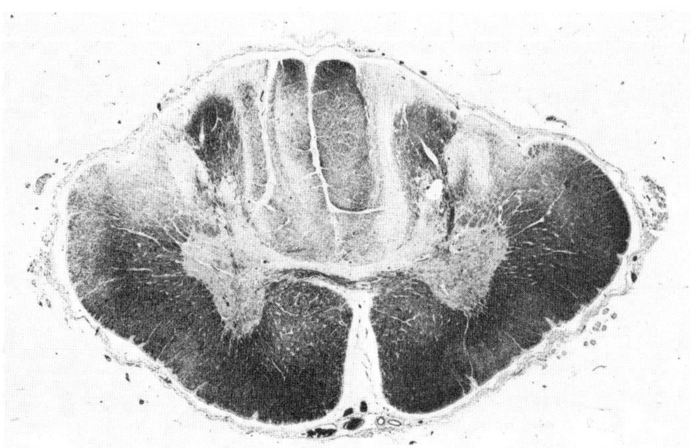

Fig. 3.14 Cervical cord (C2) × 6 showing pallor of posterior columns

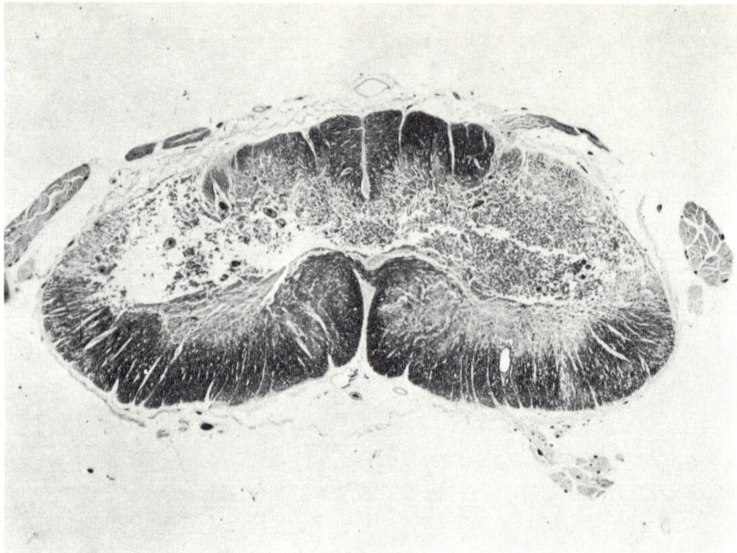

Fig. 3.15 Cervical cord (C5) × 7 showing flattening, diffuse necrosis and cavitation

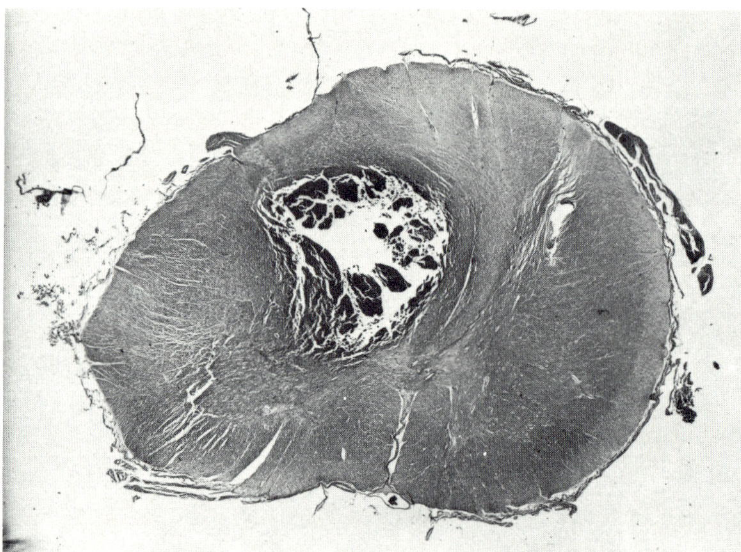

Fig. 3.16 Cervical cord (C4) × 6 showing haemorrhagic cavitation into posterior horn following an injury to the cervical spine

that all cases of myelopathy show deformity due to indentation of the spinal cord by spondylotic protrusions, although occasionally indentation of the cord may occur without there being any clinical or pathological evidence of myelopathy.

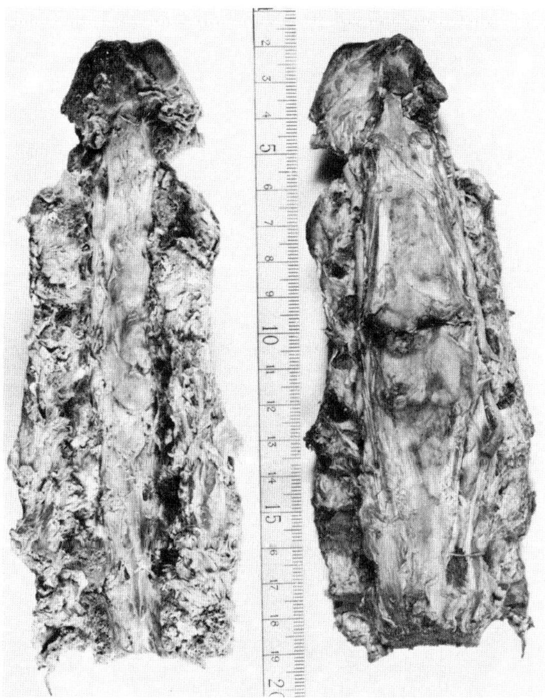

Fig. 3.17 Anterior and posterior aspects of cervical spine showing rupture of anterior ligament and haemorrhage into surrounding tissues

The Significance of Trauma in Patients with Cervical Spondylosis

The effect of trauma on patients with cervical spondylosis is usually to accentuate the already existing symptoms or to precipitate new ones. These new symptoms may be due to either root or cord lesions. In young patients acute injuries of the cervical spine may cause rupture of the annulus fibrosus with resultant prolapse of the nucleus pulposus. This prolapse may be partial or complete and the damage to the annulus fibrosus may occur at any point. Root lesions usually occur if the prolapse is lateral or postero-lateral while symptoms of cord compression can theoretically occur if the prolapse is posterior but because of the small size of the prolapse, a sphere of 0·7 cm, cord compression is unlikely in an acute disc protrusion. Spillane (1969) emphasised the way in which the presence of a congenitally small spinal canal makes a patient more subject to cord damage from a relatively minor neck injury. Such a narrow canal might also predispose a patient to cord compression from an acute disc protrusion.

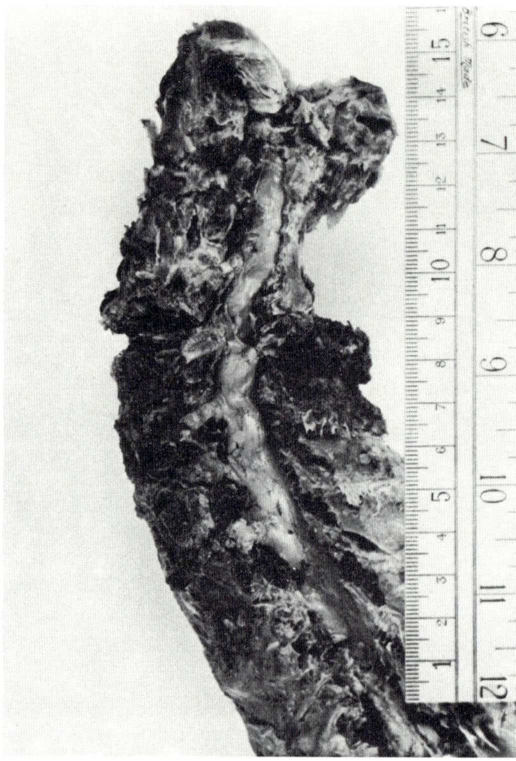

Fig. 3.18 Cervical spine with cord *in situ* showing effect of injury on the cervical cord in a case of cervical spondylosis

After acute rupture of the disc the patient may complain of severe pain in the neck with the symptoms and signs of a root lesion. The question of recurrent trauma to the neck presents a more difficult problem. In a series of 111 patients with cervical spondylosis, Wilkinson (1959) found that 52 patients (47 per cent) gave a history of having injured their neck at some time or of having had a heavy fall and of these 24 (21·5 per cent) gave a history of having had recurrent minor injuries to their necks. These recurrent injuries occurred in those whose occupations involved carrying heavy weights on their head or shoulders. Other authors give rather lower figures (Ricard and Masson 16 per cent; Brain, Northfield and Wilkinson 36 per cent and Bradshaw (1957) 22 per cent).

Damage to the cervical cord may occur if there are large spondylotic bosses or bars present. The most common acute injury to the cervical spine which causes damage to the cord is one in which the cervical spine is hyperextended (Fig. 3.17). This may be caused by a fall downstairs, a blow on the head, a "whiplash" injury sustained in a car accident or diving into shallow water. Myelopathy is also more likely if the cervical cord is tethered either by root-sleeve fibrosis or by dural adhesions particularly in those with a narrow cervical canal. Traumatic lesions of the cervical spine most commonly involve the 4th, 5th and 6th cervical vertebrae and this is probably due to the fact that the maximal convexity of the cervical lordosis is at about the level of the 5th cervical vertebrae. The cervical spine forms a solid bony column and its strength depends on the postero-lateral wall of the spinal canal, the anterior and posterior common spinal ligaments, the discs and paravertebral muscles. Dislocation of one vertebrae on the other is more likely to occur than fracture. Forcible extension may cause rupture of the anterior longitudinal ligament and where this occurs the upper vertebra may slide backwards on the lower one causing crushing of the cord (Fig. 3.18). If cervical spondylosis is present the effect of the injury is accentuated because, where there is a spondylotic boss or bar, the antero-posterior diameter of the cervical canal is already diminished and the cord may be compressed (Fig. 3.15). In such patients the dura is commonly adherent to the surrounding bone, and root-sleeve fibrosis may also be present. Because of the adhesions and root-sleeve fibrosis, the cord is firmly anchored in the cervical canal and the liability to contusion increased. Because of these factors injury to the cervical cord in patients with cervical spondylosis is common even when there is no fracture or fracture-dislocation. If the injury is not very severe the lesion may be limited to one or more nerve roots, but if cervical spondylosis is marked there may be softening of (Fig. 3.15) or haemorrhage into the cord (Fig. 3.16) with or without bony displacement. Hyperextension of the cervical spine during anaesthesia or osteopathic manipulations may cause damage to the cervical cord in patients with cervical spondylosis, especially if muscle relaxants have been given.

References

Abdullah, S. (1958), M.Sc. Thesis, London University.
Adamkiewicz, A. (1882), *S.B. Akad. Wiss. Wien (Math. Naturwiss. Kl.)*, **85**, 101.
Bedford, P. D., Bosanquet, F. D. and Russell, W. R. (1952), *Lancet,* **ii**, 55.
Biemond, A. (1951), *Brain*, **74**, 300.
Bradshaw, P. (1957), *Quart. J. Med.,* **26**, 177.

Brain, W. R. (1956), *J. Fac. Radiol.*, **8**, 74.
Brain, W. R., Northfield, D. W. C. and Wilkinson, M. (1952), *Brain*, **75**, 187.
Bull, J. W. D. (1948), *Proc. R. Soc. Med.*, **41**, 513.
Burrows, E. H. (1963), *Clin. Radiol.*, **14**, 77.
De Kleyn, A. (1939), *Confin. neurol., Basel*, **2**, 257.
De Kleyn, A. and Nieuwenheyse, P. (1927), *Acta oto-laryng., Stockh.*, **11**, 155.
Frykholm, R. (1951), *Acta chir. scand.*, suppl. **160**.
Gortvai, P. (1946), *Brit. med. J.*, **2**, 233.
Greenfield, J. G. (1953), *Rev. med. Suisse rom.*, **73**, 227.
Herren, R. Y. and Alexander, L. (1939), *Arch. Neurol. Psychiat., Chicago*, **41**, 678.
Hughes, J. T. (1966), *Pathology of the Spinal Cord*, Lloyd-Luke, London.
Hughes, J. T. and Brownell, B. (1964), *Neurology, Minneap.*, **14**, 1073.
Hutchinson, E. C. and Yates, P. O. (1956), *Brain*, **79**, 319.
Kadyi, H. (1889), *Über die Blutgefässe des menschlichen Rückenmarkes*, Gubrynowicz & Schmidt, Lemberg.
Kahn, E. A. (1947), *J. Neurosurg.*, **4**, 191.
Krogdahl, T. and Torgerson, O. (1940), *Acta radiol., Stockh.*, **21**, 231.
Love, J. G. and Walsh, M. N. (1940), *Arch. Surg.*, **40**, 454.
Lowman, R. M. and Finkelstein, A. (1942), *Radiology*, **39**, 700.
Mair, W. G. P. and Druckman, R. (1953), *Brain*, **76**, 70.
Pallis, C. A., Jones, A. M. and Spillane, J. D. (1954), *Brain*, **77**, 274.
Payne, E. E. and Spillane, J. D. (1957), *Brain*, **80**, 571.
Petter, C. K. (1933), *J. Bone Jt. Surg.*, **15**, 365.
Püschel, J. (1930), *Beitr. path. Anat.*, **84**, 123.
Ricard, A. and Masson, R. (1951), *Rev. neurol.*, **85**, 420.
Saunders, J. B. de C. M. and Inman, V. T. (1939), *Int. Abstr. Surg.*, **69**, 14.
Sheehan, S., Bauer, R. B. and Meyer, J. S. (1960), *Neurology, Minneap.*, **10**, 968.
Spillane, J. D. (1969), personal communication.
Stoltmann, H. F. and Blackwood, W. (1964), *Brain*, **87**, 45.
Tatlow, W. F. T. and Bammer, H. G. (1957), *Neurology, Minneap.*, **7**, 331.
Taylor, A. R. (1951), *J. Bone Jt. Surg.*, **33B**, 543.
Taylor, A. R. (1964), *Neurology, Minneap.*, **14**, 62.
Virtama, P. and Kivalo, E. (1957), *Acta radiol., Stockh.*, **48**, 410.
Wilkinson, M. (1959), "Cervical Spondylosis" (DM Thesis, Oxford University).
Wilkinson, M. (1960), *Brain*, **83**, 589.
Wolf, B. S., Khilnani, M. and Malis, L. (1956), *J. Mt. Sinai Hosp.*, **23**, 283.

Chapter IV

Symptomatology

Marcia Wilkinson

The symptoms and signs of cervical spondylosis fall into two main groups, those due to root compression—cervical radiculopathy, and those due to cord compression—cervical myelopathy. In addition there may be other related symptoms which include headache, pain in the neck and the symptoms of vertebro-basilar insufficiency. All these may occur singly or in any combination.

1. CERVICAL RADICULOPATHY

In cervical spondylosis root involvement may be single or multiple, unilateral or bilateral, symmetrical or asymmetrical, and the degree of involvement of each particular root is variable. Not uncommonly root involvement is associated with cord involvement. Three main types of radiculopathy can be distinguished.

(a) Acute Radiculopathy

In an injury there may be a tear of the annulus fibrosus with consequent prolapse of the nucleus pulposus. The resulting neurological picture depends on the site of the lesion. An acute dorso-lateral disc protrusion may compress the root against the vertebral lamina or an acute intraforaminal protrusion may compress the radicular nerve against the articular process, the intraforaminal protrusion coming from the uncinate part of the disc. These lesions may occur in patients in whom there is little or no evidence of pre-existing spondylosis but who have received some injury to the neck, such as a blow or in a fall. Characteristically these patients are young.

There is a second group in whom an acute disc protrusion or an exacerbation of a pre-existing protrusion may occur in association with spondylotic changes which X-rays show to be of long standing. In these patients also there is often a history of trauma and it is probable that the pathology is the same as that of the first group, with a rupture of the annulus fibrosus and protrusion of the nucleus pulposus.

Sometimes the symptoms of acute radiculopathy do not entirely subside but leave some permanent sensory disturbances—usually pain. In some the symptoms of a chronic radiculopathy develop insidiously.

(b) Subacute Radiculopathy

This is the classical "brachial neuritis" which may occur in patients with cervical spondylosis and here it appears that the pathology may be different. There is no history of acute trauma and it is possible that there is no acute disc prolapse. The patient has had radiological evidence of cervical spondylosis for years, perhaps with no symptoms except occasional pain in the neck and he then develops acutely or sub-acutely a radiculopathy which may involve one or more roots. In these patients repeated mild trauma or an unidentified inflammatory process may be responsible for the radicular symptoms. In the majority of cases the symptoms clear up over about 6 weeks particularly if the patient can rest and analgesics are given.

(c) Chronic Radiculopathy

The symptoms of a chronic radiculopathy may develop insidiously or the symptoms and signs may not clear up after an acute attack and the pain lingers on. One of the commonest complaints of middle-aged or elderly patients is pain in the neck or arm especially if they do heavy work to which they are not accustomed. Many middle-aged and elderly people do heavy work only intermittently and it is these who are particularly liable to get "brachial neuritis". Very often women develop symptoms as the result of carrying heavy shopping baskets, and where this is a precipitating feature the use of a trolley will often cause improvement. Other occupations likely to precipitate an attack of radiculopathy are gardening or household decorating, particularly if the ceilings are being done. Painting a ceiling involves not only heavy work above shoulder level but also hyperextension of the neck and both these factors may play a part in the precipitation of symptoms.

SYMPTOMS—SIGNS OF RADICULOPATHY

(a) Acute Radiculopathy

Sensory symptoms are far more frequent than motor and the most common irritative root symptom is pain although various forms of paraesthesiae, hyperaesthesia and hyperalgesia may occur. Less commonly there are reflex and motor changes.

(i) Sensory symptoms and signs

In acute radiculopathy the onset of pain begins quite suddenly a few minutes or hours after the trauma and reaches its maximum within a few days. It is a severe aching or shooting pain and its distribution is radicular corresponding to that of the cervical nerve root involved. Since each spinal nerve supplies pain sensitivity to bones, joints, muscles and blood vessels as well as skin over a wide area it follows that even when only one nerve root is affected the pain irradiates widely—characteristically into the neck and shoulders and down the arm and forearm to the digits receiving the nerve supply from the particular root or roots affected. It may also extend into the chest both anteriorly and posteriorly especially when the 5th, 6th or 7th cervical nerve root is involved.

The pain is often modified by the position of the neck, which itself is painful and the site of muscular spasm. It may be made worse by active or passive rotation, tilting, flexion or extension of the head and often by lying on the affected side; usually the most comfortable position is the supine one with the head slightly flexed on the trunk. Unlike the pain of sciatica it is not usually exacerbated by coughing.

In this type of brachial radiculopathy other sensory symptoms and signs are less prominent than pain although there may be numbness and tingling within the dermatome innervated by the affected root associated with some impairment of cutaneous sensibility.

(ii) Muscular weakness

In a proportion of patients with an acute radiculopathy severe muscular weakness may occur. This occurs in patients in whom there has been an acute prolapse of the nucleus pulposus usually either posterolateral or intraforaminal, which has caused direct compression of the nerve root. The onset is acute and is usually associated with pain of the kind described above. But coincident with the pain or in the space of a few hours the patient notices that his arm has become very weak. This is due to involvement of the motor as well as the sensory root, the 5th and 6th cervical roots being the ones most commonly affected, and the distribution of the muscular weakness corresponds to the motor supply of the nerve root involved. When this is the 5th cervical, the spinati, deltoid, biceps, brachio-radialis and the supinator are the most affected. In the case of the 6th cervical root the muscles involved are the triceps, pectoralis major, latissimus dorsi and extensors of the wrists. Wasting of the affected muscles rapidly develops, sometimes associated with fasciculation, and the appropriate tendon reflexes are diminished or lost.

(b) Symptoms of Subacute Radiculopathy

In the classical "brachial neuritis" pain is again a prominent symptom and may be as severe as in an acute radiculopathy. It may be limited to the distribution of a single root or may be more extensive as often more than one root may be involved. The pain may be referred to the neck and sometimes there is an associated muscular spasm. Dysaesthesiae, i.e. unpleasant sensations of numbness or tingling, are common especially in the digits corresponding to the root or roots involved. It is most important to take an accurate history from these patients because the distribution of pain and/or dysaesthesiae may be the only indication of the root or roots involved. Often there is slight muscular wasting and hypotonia but pronounced muscular weakness is uncommon. As the 6th or 7th cervical roots are the ones most frequently involved, the triceps is the muscle most often affected. The appropriate tendon reflexes are diminished or absent. A frozen shoulder (p. 151) is a common complication.

2. CERVICAL MYELOPATHY

In cervical myelopathy there is ischaemia or compression of the spinal cord by the spondylotic bosses and bars and surrounding structures. The changes in the spinal cord are produced in a complex fashion by the pressures and tensions to which it is subjected. Since these changes are the result of a number of variables it is easy to understand why there should be great variability in the resulting clinical picture. The causal lesion may be a single osteophyte which may compress the spinal cord at any point between the upper and lower limits of the cervical enlargement, or there may be two or more such osteophytes at different levels. Moreover at any one particular level the extent to which the grey and white matter are affected, and, within the white matter, the anterior, lateral and posterior columns, is very variable. As a result of this the resulting clinical picture is usually that of an incomplete lesion of the spinal cord involving particular elements in a patchy manner, sometimes limited to a single segmental level, but often involving several levels to a greater or lesser extent. Because of this a description will be given of what may be called an average case and an account of the more exceptional manifestations will be given later.

Myelopathy of Insidious Onset

The Average Clinical Picture

In cervical myelopathy the onset is usually insidious, the patient complaining of increasing disability over a period of months. Very often there is also a history of radicular symptoms, for example an attack of brachial neuritis. The three common initial symptoms which may occur alone or in combination are dysaesthesiae in the hands, weakness and clumsiness of the hands and weakness of the lower limbs.

(a) Sensory symptoms and signs

The dysaesthesiae consist of numbness and tingling, especially in the tips of the digits, often of radicular distribution, for example in the thumb and index finger when the 6th cervical segment is mainly involved. Very often the symptoms of radiculopathy and myelopathy co-exist and this complicates the clinical picture. If radiculopathy is present there may be pain of radicular distribution. Gross impairment of sensation is not a feature of the average clinical picture. Usually there is some impairment of appreciation of light touch, tactile discrimination and pinprick over some or all of the digits of the hands, and this sometimes extends upwards, especially on the radial border of the forearm, and it is frequently asymmetrical. Occasionally cutaneous sensory loss extends on the upper limbs or neck one or two dermatomes above the upper segmental level of the spinal compression. In the lower limbs there may also be some areas of impairment of appreciation of pain, heat and cold. Vibration sense is often impaired or lost below the iliac crest or costal margins, and there may be some impairment over the digits of the upper limbs. Appreciation of passive movement in the fingers and toes is usually normal or slightly impaired.

(b) Motor symptoms and signs

Weakness and clumsiness may be present in one or both hands. The degree of wasting in the upper limbs is very variable both in extent and severity, its distribution depending upon the segments of cord involved. When these occupy the upper part of the cervical enlargement muscular wasting is likely to occur in the spinati, deltoid, biceps, triceps and pectoralis major. The dorsiflexors of the wrists and fingers may also be affected. When the lower part of the cervical enlargement is the main site of the disorder, the brunt of the wasting will fall upon the flexors of the wrist and fingers and the small muscles of the hand. The wasting may be slight or severe with a corresponding degree of weakness. In cervical myelopathy there is cortico-spinal tract involvement below the level of the lesion while if there is a co-existing motor radiculopathy the signs will be those of a lower motor neurone lesion of that segment.

Muscle fasciculation is usually inconspicuous and if it does occur is generally of segmental distribution. In other cases a little flickering can be observed in a wasted muscle particularly in the triceps. Although the fasciculation is never so severe or widespread as seen in advanced cases of motor neurone disease, in some patients it may be enough to present diagnostic difficulties.

In the lower limbs the most usual clinical picture is that of a spastic weakness, one leg often being rather more severely affected than the other. Slight general wasting, as is common in paraplegia, is likely to be present. Very rarely more conspicuous wasting, sometimes with fasciculation, may be observed in the lower limbs. The cause of this is uncertain but it may be related to interference with the blood supply of the lower part of the cord. Muscular wasting and pain in the lower limbs may be due to an associated lumbar spondylosis.

(c) The tendon reflexes

The tendon reflexes are often of considerable diagnostic importance. It is important that the jaw jerk should be tested since a normal jaw jerk associated with exaggerated tendon reflexes in the upper limbs is strongly suggestive of a lesion below the foramen magnum, whereas an exaggerated jaw jerk indicates the possibility of a lesion above the level of the pons.

The tendon reflexes in the upper limbs will depend upon a balance of two factors, the upper and lower motor neurone lesions. Involvement of anterior horn cells, and hence the lower motor neurones, in the myelopathy will tend to diminish and ultimately abolish the tendon reflexes involving that spinal segment. On the other hand involvement of the cortico-spinal tracts will produce exaggeration of the tendon reflexes. Hence when the cervical enlargement itself is spared but there is a disc protrusion involving the cord just above it, all the tendon jerks in the upper limbs will be exaggerated. When, as is usually the case, the cervical enlargement itself is involved, there will often be a combination of diminution of some tendon reflexes with exaggeration of others. The triceps jerk is the one most commonly diminished or lost owing to the frequency with which the 6th segment is involved.

One of the most characteristic changes in the reflexes in the upper limb in cervical spondylosis is the so-called "inverted radial reflex". This results from involvement of the 5th cervical segment, through which pass most of the nervous pathways concerned in the radial reflex. When a lesion of this segment also involves the cortico-spinal tract it is likely to cause exaggeration of the tendon reflexes mediated by lower segments of the cervical cord, particularly the flexor finger jerk. The consequence is that on percussing the lower end of the radius, the normal radial reflex is much diminished or lost, but the stimulus by irradiation evokes reflex flexion of the digits. This combination is called the "inverted radial reflex". The exaggeration of flexor finger jerks can always be demonstrated by percussing the flexor aspects of the digits directly, or by means of Hoffmann's reflex. The triceps jerk also is often exaggerated in these cases and there are upper motor neurone signs in the lower limbs. The inverted radial reflex is by no means always present in cervical myelopathy due to spondylosis, so its absence does not exclude that diagnosis. Nor, on the other hand, is it pathognomonic, for it may be encountered with other cord lesions, provided that they selectively involve the 5th cervical segment.

The abdominal reflexes are usually diminished, but rarely completely lost. This is a useful diagnostic point as patients with disseminated sclerosis characteristically lose the abdominal reflexes early in their disease. The spasticity of the lower limbs produces exaggeration of the knee and ankle jerks, sometimes with clonus; and the plantar reflexes are likely to be extensor.

One of the conspicuous features of the average clinical picture in cervical spondylosis is the absence of impairment of sphincter control.

Less Common Clinical Pictures

The less common clinical pictures are important because they may not be recognised as due to cervical spondylosis, and may be confused with those of other disorders.

Exceptionally, the symptoms are motor only, being characterised by muscular wasting in the upper limbs and spastic weakness of the lower limbs, a clinical picture which may closely simulate motor neurone disease. Very rarely the cortico-spinal tracts are exclusively affected, resulted in a clinical picture resembling that described in the past as "primary lateral sclerosis". Exceptionally, again, the symptoms may be limited to the lower limbs, presenting purely as a spastic paraplegia with no detectable symptoms or signs in the upper limbs.

Occasionally, posterior column sensibility suffers severely, and always in association with some of the other symptoms and signs described as part of the average clinical picture. The addition to this of gross impairment of postural sensibility in the upper and lower limbs causes a great increase in the disability. The resulting clinical picture may simulate subacute combined degeneration. An important diagnostic point is the frequency with which a segmental level for the upper limit of impaired postural sensibility can be demonstrated in the digits of the upper limb, for example, there may be sparing of the thumb or thumb and index finger when there is gross impairment of appreciation of passive movement in the middle, ring and little fingers.

Finally, there is the clinical picture of the advanced stages of the disorder when the patient is bedridden with severe paraplegia or quadriplegia, a variable degree of sensory loss, and, at this stage, impairment of sphincter control.

The cerebrospinal fluid

The composition of the cerebrospinal fluid in cervical spondylosis is usually normal: exceptionally there is a rise in the protein content but this is usually not above 80–100 mg per cent unless there is marked cord compression. There is no excess of cells and the colloidal gold curve is normal. If in the course of a lumbar puncture to estimate the pressure of the fluid, the patient's head is in the normal position, the neck being neither flexed nor extended, the pressure of the fluid will be normal and there will be a normal rise and fall in the course of Queckenstedt's test. In some cases of cervical spondylosis with signs of cord involvement it has been shown that if the neck is passively extended there will be some impairment of the rate of rise and fall of the fluid, i.e. a partial but not complete block.

Myelopathy of Acute or Subacute Onset

1. Subacute onset due to spontaneous subluxation

Occasionally the symptoms of cervical myelopathy develop rapidly, and become severe in the course of a few weeks. This is liable to happen when degeneration of an intervertebral disc allows abnormal movement to occur between the body of one vertebra and that of the one immediately below it. Usually the upper body moves forwards, but sometimes the degree of abnormal mobility is so great that when X-rays are taken with the head erect, in flexion and in extension, the upper body may be seen to move forwards in flexion and backwards in extension. Apart from its rapidity of onset, the clinical picture does not differ greatly from that of the chronic form of cervical myelopathy, but on the whole there is a tendency for all the long tracts of the spinal cord to be involved. Radicular symptoms may precede or accompany those of the myelopathy. Although the onset of symptoms is subacute, the X-ray changes of cervical spondylosis in these cases are of long standing and it seems likely that the subluxation occurs gradually and only when it reaches a certain point do symptoms come on rapidly.

2. Acute onset due to a superimposed vascular lesion

This is a rare occurrence, and is usually seen in patients with hypertension or other evidence of cardiovascular disease. There may or may not have been previous symptoms of cervical spondylosis. The vascular lesion, probably ischaemic, usually involves a sector of the cord on one side at the level of the degenerated intervertebral disc.

3. Acute onset due to trauma

In a patient who has cervical spondylosis, an injury to the head or neck may produce immediate and severe symptoms. Extension of the neck seems the most important aetiological factor, and may be produced in a variety of ways. It may follow any severe blow on the front of the head or a "whiplash injury" resulting from a motor-car accident. Another cause of symptoms is vigorous extension of the neck in the course of surgical operations or the preliminary anaesthetic procedures. The resulting symptoms may be either those of an acute myelopathy ranging in severity from severe quadriplegia to a mild incomplete lesion of the spinal cord at the cervical level, or an acute brachial radiculopathy which may be either unilateral or bilateral, and involve one or more spinal roots, and again, may be either mild or severe.

3. PAIN IN THE NECK

Since it is the cervical spine which is responsible for all the symptoms of cervical spondylosis, it might be thought that the neck itself would commonly be a site of symptoms, but symptoms referred to the neck in cervical spondylosis are as often slight or absent as they are present. Quite severe radiographic changes in the cervical spine may be unassociated with any neck symptoms.

Pain in the neck in cervical spondylosis may be produced in several ways. An acute disc protrusion is likely to be associated with severe pain, muscular spasm, and rigidity. Such an acute protrusion may have been preceded by brief attacks of less severe pain, not uncommonly labelled "fibrositis". In chronic cervical spondylosis pain is only rarely severe. It is usually comparatively mild, and tends to be worse when the patient awakens in the morning. It may be made worse by active and passive movements, which may be associated with crepitus, sometimes audible both to the patient and to the observer. A painful neck in cervical spondylosis is often tender on deep pressure over the cervical muscles or over one or more spinous processes.

Active and passive movements of the cervical spine are often somewhat limited and may be severely so: on the other hand, it is sometimes surprising how full such movements are in view of the radiographic appearances of severe changes. Passive movements of the neck may cause pain to be referred to one or other shoulder and, when brachial radiculopathy is present, down the arm also. Conversely, the pain in a brachial radiculopathy may be temporarily relieved by traction on the cervical spine.

4. HEADACHE

Headache is a fairly common symptom of cervical spondylosis. Its pathogenesis is still not fully understood. Characteristically it is located in the occiput on one or both sides and may be described as spreading through the parieto-temporal region to the frontal region and the eye. It tends to be worse on awakening in the morning and to pass off during the day. This type of headache may occur when the spondylotic changes involve the lower cervical discs, as well as when the upper apophyseal joints are involved.

5. VERTEBRO-BASILAR INSUFFICIENCY

Cervical spondylosis may affect the cerebral circulation because of the anatomical relationship between the vertebral arteries and the cervical spine. It will be remembered that the vertebral arteries enter the cervical spine at the level of the 6th cervical vertebra, and pass upwards through a canal in the transverse processes. Emerging from the transverse process of the atlas, they loop round to enter the skull through the foramen magnum. Within the cervical spine, therefore, the vertebral arteries are closely related to the neurocentral joints medially, and the zygapophyseal joints postero-laterally. The two arteries are often markedly unequal in size.

Certain physiological and pathological factors may influence the blood flow through the vertebral arteries. There is angiographic evidence that even in normal people rotation of the head to one side may temporarily impair the blood flow through the vertebral artery, on the side towards which the head is turned, in its course between the 6th and 7th cervical vertebrae, and in the opposite vertebral artery, where it passes through the transverse process of the atlas. Such temporary circulatory changes produce no symptoms in normal people because of the provision of anastomotic channels from the internal carotid arteries by the circle of Willis. If the blood flow to the circle of Willis is temporarily impaired through one of its contributory vessels the direction of the circulation within the circle itself changes, so that the deficiency is supplied from the remaining channels.

Hutchinson and Yates (1956) have shown that even when the head is in the normal position, one or both vertebral arteries may be considerably distorted and narrowed by osteophytes derived from the neurocentral and apophyseal joints. This effect is enhanced by head rotation as just described. The same authors have shown that when both carotids and both vertebral arteries are atheromatous, the efficiency of the collateral circulation through the circle of Willis just described, is impaired, and further narrowing of one vessel, for example, one internal carotid artery by thrombosis, may impair the blood supply to the brain structures normally supplied by the vertebral arteries, and may thus even lead to infarction of the cerebellum. It is the combination of cervical spondylosis with atheroma in the vertebral arteries, especially if one or both carotids are also narrowed, that is most productive of ischaemic symptoms.

The characteristic feature is of precipitation of paroxysmal symptoms by head movement, often rotation to one or other side or extension of the neck, and, less frequently, flexion. Such movements may precipitate a brief attack of giddiness, diplopia or a drop attack, in which the patient suddenly falls without impairment of consciousness, or an attack of syncope. Each of these symptoms, however, may occur spontaneously in the absence of head movement, in patients suffering from vertebro-basilar ischaemia.

Strokes due to persistent ischaemia within the vertebro-basilar distribution may also occur in patients with vertebral artery atheroma and cervical spondylosis. Cases are on record in which such persistent ischaemic lesions have been precipitated by manipulation of the neck.

Reference

Hutchinson, E. C. and Yates, P. O. (1956), *Brain*, **79**, 319.

Chapter V

Radiology of the Cervical Spine

ALLAN C. YOUNG

Although this chapter deals with cervical spondylosis in detail this common degenerative condition is viewed in relation to other disorders which the physician may encounter during clinical practice. It is necessary for him or her to be able to request appropriate X-ray views and in some cases to request special examinations. In order that the clinician may be able to make an assessment of the appearances, it has been thought worthwhile to discuss in some detail the radiography of the cervical spine and then the normal appearances of the films taken during the routine examinations. The movements of the cervical spine may be particularly important and these are analysed at some length.

A recognition of the abnormal depends upon a knowledge of the normal, and normal films have been included to act as a base line for the study of clinical examples by the clinician who has very many other things to do apart from looking at X-ray films. The best results in radiology are usually achieved by close co-operation between the clinician, the radiographer and the radiologist. It is in the belief that the more a clinician can bring to a conference, the more he and his radiological colleagues can gain from it, that technical matters are considered in some depth.

RADIOGRAPHY

(ANN PARIS)

A detailed examination should demonstrate all the 23 articulations of the cervical spine and the way in which they move, especially in flexion and extension. Patients with bad necks are difficult to examine and a full examination of the cervical spine may be a lengthy business, perhaps taking up to $1\frac{1}{2}$ hours or more. It is worth considering that it might be in everyone's interest to give the patient a specific appointment in the X-ray department rather than put up with indifferent results which are so often the outcome of a routine job.

Apparatus

The generator should have an output of 400 mA at 65–75 kV thus allowing short exposure times; a fine-focus (0·6 mm) tube should be fitted to give good detail on the radiograph. The use of fast films with fast or standard screens reduces irradiation but fast films used with high definition screens will ensure a better result.

A wall mounted Bucky stand which can be used in the vertical or horizontal position enables patient to be examined standing, seated or on a non-opaque stretcher. A head clamp should be available. The examination is made easier if an adjustable chair is available; this should have the following movements: elevation and depression; rotation; forward, backward and sideways movement. It should be possible to adjust it quickly and without too much effort, and when the desired position has been achieved it must be maintained by an efficient locking device.

Oblique and antero-posterior (A.P.) films should always have both left and right sides clearly marked; all views, except the antero-posterior views, should be taken with a tube–film distance of 6 in. to minimise magnification.

Available Standard Views (Fig. 5.1)

(1) Antero-posterior (A.P.) (Fig. 5.1a). C3 to C7, tube angled 10 degrees up, occiput and lower jaw superimposed; central ray C4. This view demonstrates posture, the neurocentral joints and the lateral masses. It is essential for the demonstration of congenital anomalies but it shows only gross degenerative changes in the zygapophyseal joints.

(2) Lateral (Fig. 5.1b)—chin half extended, central ray C3. This shows the general posture of the spine, the height of the discs, anterior and posterior osteophytosis, the superimposed zygapophyseal joints, the laminae and spinous processes. It enables the discs and the antero-posterior diameter of the cervical canal to be measured.

(3 and 4) Oblique views (Fig. 1c and d). The intervertebral foramen is more of a canal than a simple opening. Coliez (1965) likens it to "une gargouille", the water spout from which our "gargoyle" is derived (Fig. 5.2). He points out that the transverse canal is directed downwards and posteriorly. In order to demonstrate this completely the patient should be turned 50 degrees from the A.P. position and the central ray angled 10 degrees upwards centred at C3. Although the zygapophyseal joints are not fully demonstrated in this view encroachment upon the foramina by the zygapophyseal osteophytes will be shown (Fig. 5.1b).

(5 and 6) "Off lateral" views (Fig. 5.3a and b)—in order to demonstrate zygapophyseal joint changes a supplementary view has been devised by Paris and Young (1967). A post-mortem specimen of the cervical spine was X-rayed in different degrees of obliquity. The angles used were 6, 8, 10, 12 and 14 degrees of deviation from the true lateral position. Films taken at 12 and 14 degrees and some of those taken at 10 degrees show the zygapophyseal joints in profile and separated by a wide enough margin to enable them to be distinguished. After trials with patients it was decided that 12 degrees would give the most reliable results. The example shown (Fig. 5.3a and b) demonstrates the value of this view. As the zygapophyseal joints are almost co-planar and have mildly curved surfaces both "off lateral" views should be taken in order to obtain most information.

(7 and 8) Lateral views in flexion and extension (Fig. 5.1e and f). These are of value for demonstrating normal variation, true subluxation and even dislocation which may be shown only in full flexion after trauma.

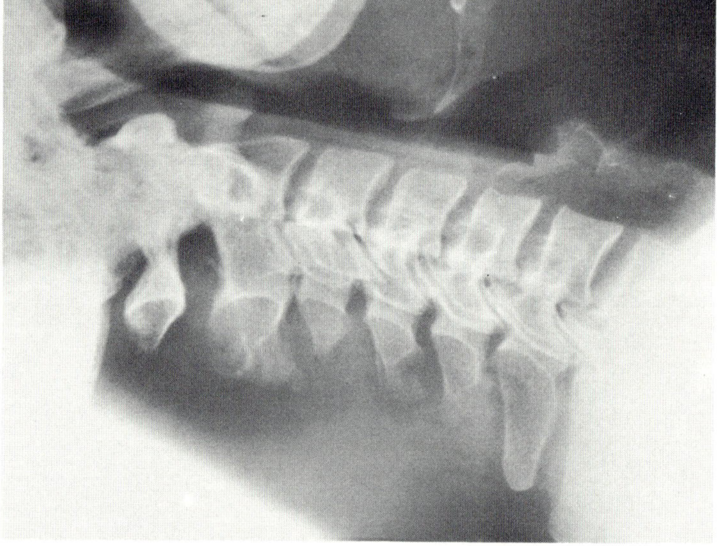

Fig. 5.1b

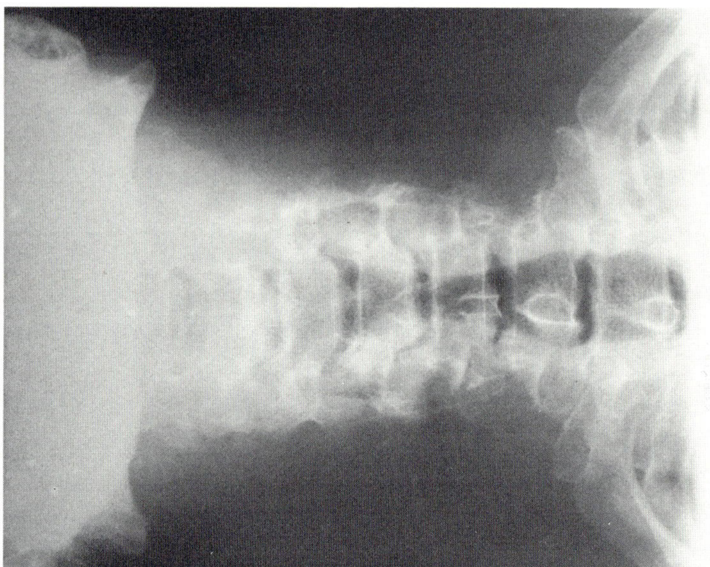

Fig. 5.1a

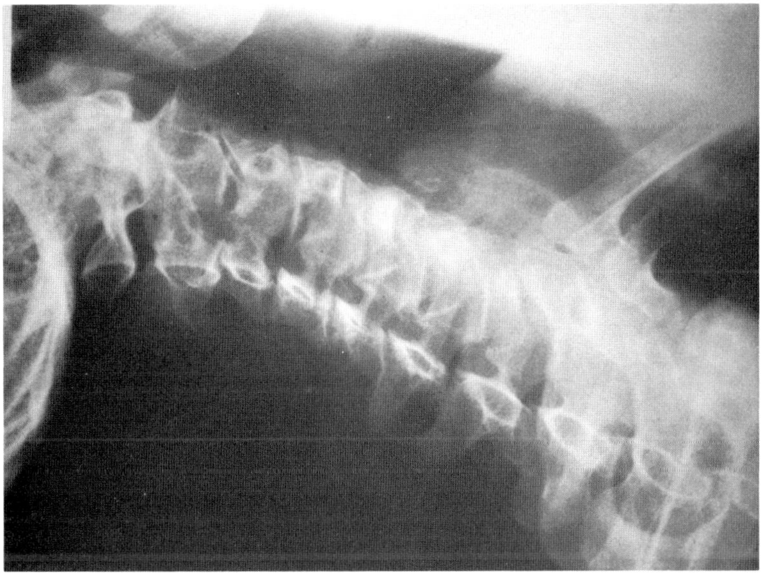

Fig. 5.1d

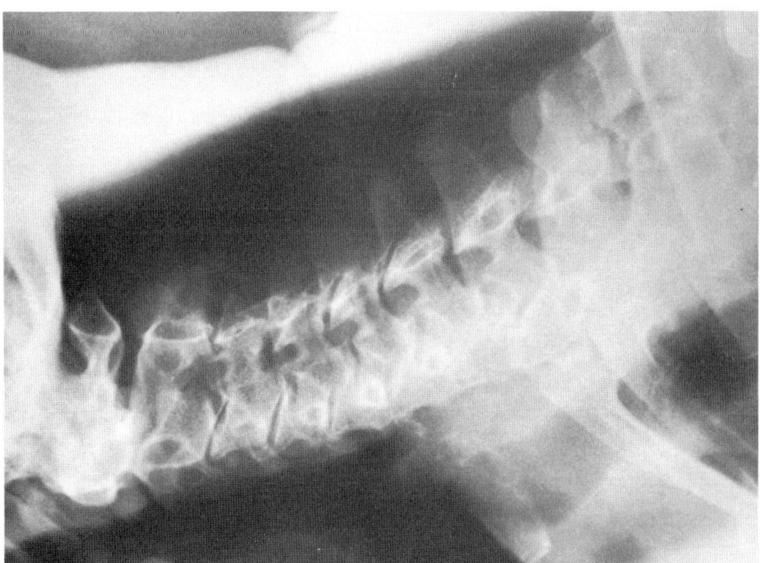

Fig. 5.1c

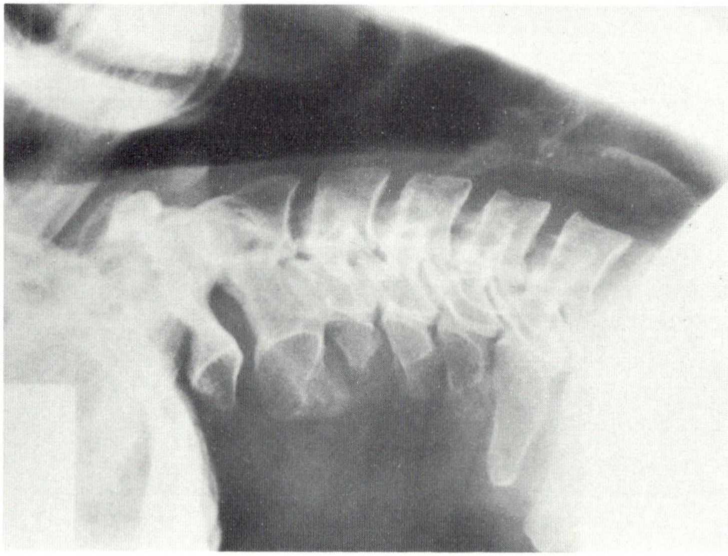

Fig. 5.1f

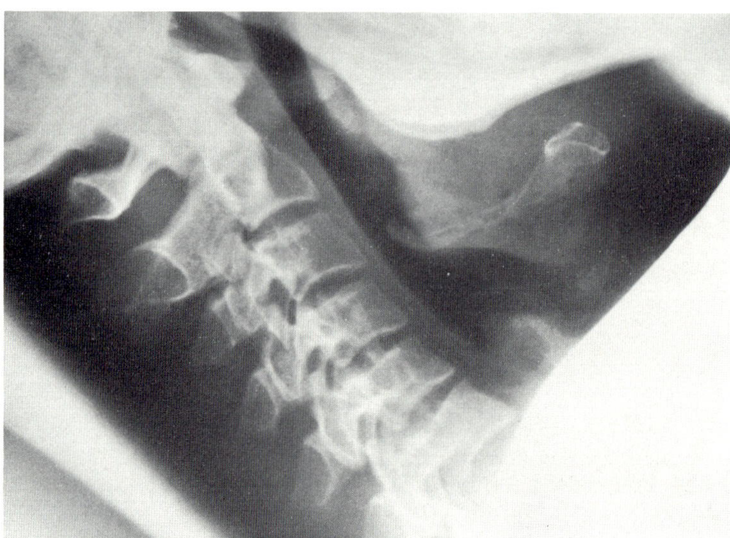

Fig. 5.1e

(9) Antero-posterior view of the atlanto-axial joints (Fig. 5.1g)—Radiographic base line (English) tilted 25 degrees up so that the occiput is superimposed upon the hard palate; central ray through middle of wide open mouth. Alternatively the teeth can be "blurred out" by taking the film while the lower jaw is moving: if this method is used the whole cervical spine from C1–C7 can be visualised.

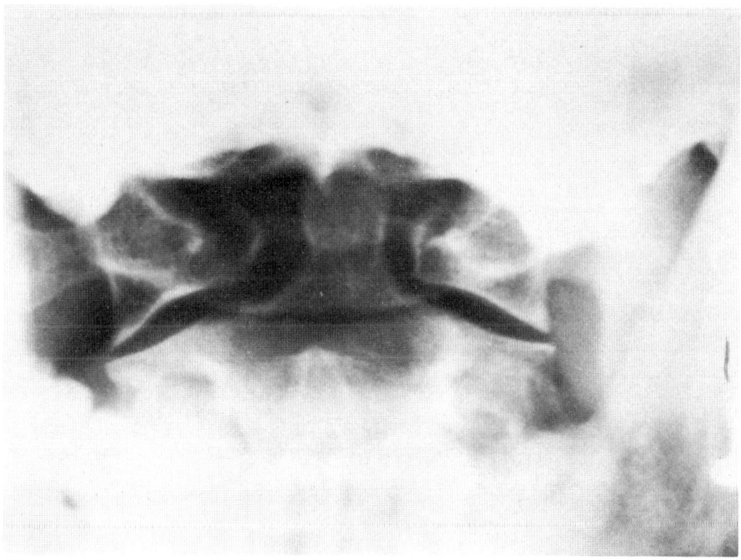

Fig. 5.1g

This view completes the A.P. visualisation of the cervical spine. It shows the odontoid process, and lower lateral articulations of the atlas.

(10 and 11) A.P. views with lateral flexion may give additional information about function (Brain, 1963).

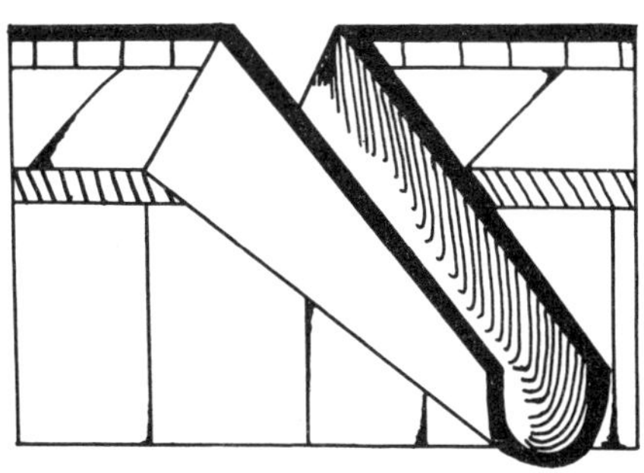

Fig. 5.2 This is "une gargouille"

(12) Autotomography of the odontoid process—patient supine, X-ray beam horizontal; patient is asked to shake his head as if saying "no" slowly and evenly; each "shake" to rotate the head 5 degrees either side of the midline. In order to assess basilar invagination this view must include the occiput. It is valuable in the detection of erosive lesions of rheumatoid arthritis and ankylosing spondylitis.

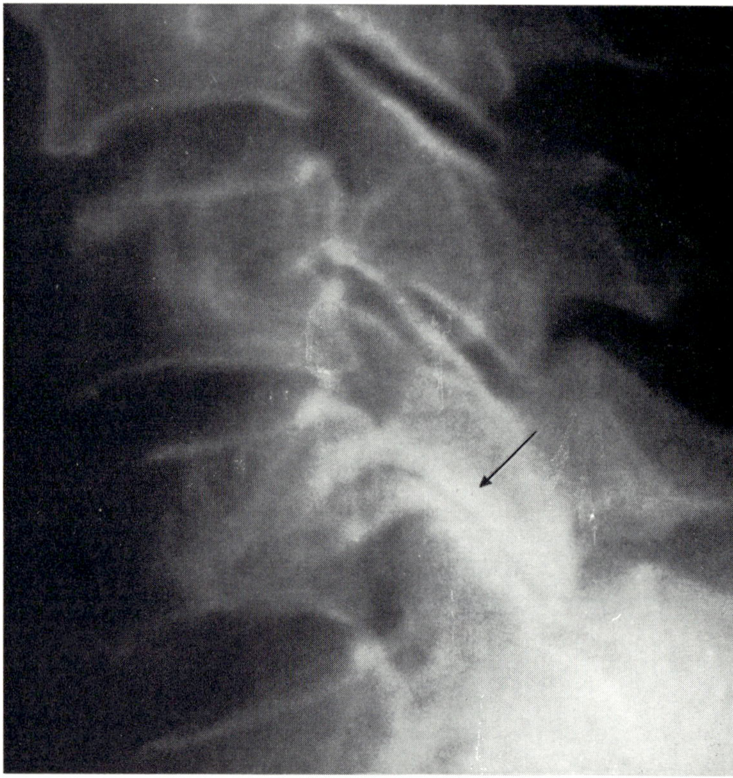

Fig. 5.3a There is obviously gross zygapophyseal arthrosis. Is it bilateral or unilateral?

(13 and 14) Rotation views of the atlanto-axial joints—patient in the A.P. position as for the odontoid peg. The radiographer places her forefinger in the notch of the thyroid cartilage and the patient turns the head until the larynx is about to move. This ensures that the rotation is confined to the atlanto-axial joint.

When the head is turned to the right the left lateral mass of the atlas is seen to move up to 5 mm medially on the lateral mass of the axis. The lateral masses on the right side remain co-linear. When the head is turned to the left the reverse conditions apply. This method occasionally gives additional evidence of rheumatoid arthritis and ankylosing spondylitis.

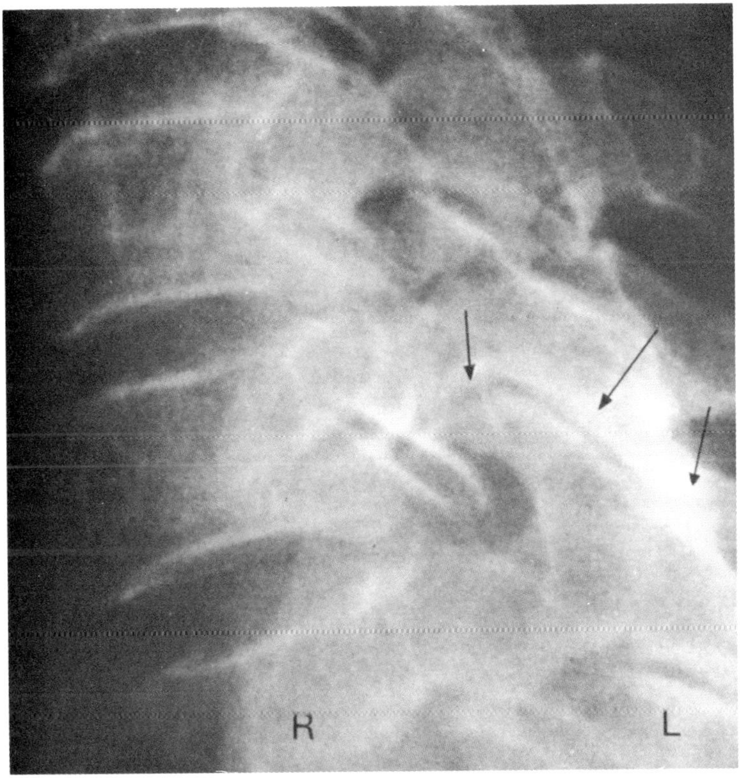

Fig. 5.3b The off lateral view shows that it is the left zygapophyseal joint which is abnormal. The anterior osteophytes are hooked and thus prevent subluxation

Special techniques

(1) Tomography This may be applied in the A.P. lateral or oblique planes. It is useful for demonstrating the precise location of osteophytes and is essential in pneumomyelography (q.v). It is also used in other conditions including primary and secondary neoplasms and congenital lesions. It gives more precise information about the atlanto-odontoid articulation (Fig. 5.11) than automography, but it takes longer to perform, and needs more complex apparatus.

(2) Myelography Two methods are available for cervical myelography; positive contrast, using an iodine containing non-soluble substance (Myodil is the same as

Pantopaque, and both are more correctly known as ethyl iodophenyl-undecanoate B.C.P. and U.S.P.), and negative contrast using gas (pneumomyelography, q.v.). Positive contrast myelography will be described first, and is the only method illustrated pictorially. Water soluble contrast media can be lethal in the cervical spine and must not be allowed to touch the cord. The use of water soluble media is therefore strictly confined to the lumbar region.

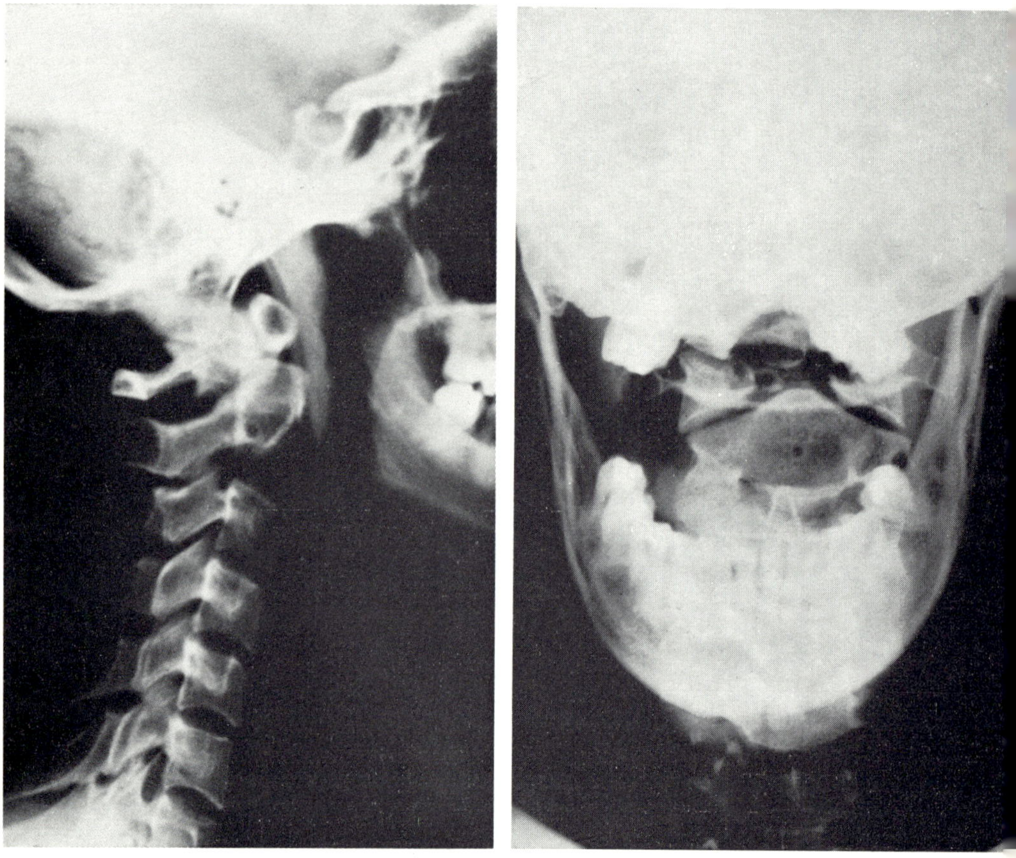

Fig. 5.4 Congenital separation of odontoid with backward dislocation

(A) Positive contrast myelography

Ideally the radiographic apparatus should include a table which tilts 90 degrees in both directions. It is possible to carry out myelography on a table which tilts 90 degrees in one direction and 15 degrees in another, but this involves rotating the patient during the examination, making the operation difficult and time consuming. As well as the usual screen and spot film device, there must be a film holder to enable lateral films to be taken with the horizontal beam.

It is unwise to perform myelography within 2 weeks of a lumbar puncture because of the possibility of a subdural leak.

The patient should be premedicated and reassured. Myodil may be introduced via the lumbar or cisternal route. If there is evidence of complete block in the spinal canal, then its upper limit will only be shown from above. But since this is rare in un complicated cervical spondylosis, the lumbar route is generally used. Lumbar puncture is carried out in the left lateral position, or in the sitting position, depending upon the preference of the examiner. The cerebrospinal fluid must flow freely; if there is any doubt, 1 ml Myodil can be injected and watched under the fluoroscopic screen; if it moves freely the needle is in a satisfactory position. A truly mid-line tap is essential; A.P. and lateral films of the lumbar spine should be taken first so as to warn the examiner of scoliosis and other difficulties.

Although 5–6 ml of Myodil is generally advocated, the diagnosis of cervical spondylosis requires a larger volume. This is because lesions are often multiple and extend over a long distance. James (1965) suggests that 12–24 ml is a reasonable amount. In order to examine the cervical region fully the Myodil must be seen up to cisterna magna.

Authorities vary as to whether Myodil should be left in the subarachnoid space after myelography. Grainger (1960) implies that its removal is not usually necessary. If a large volume is used it is easier to remove, and presumably a large volume is more likely to produce arachnoiditis. It seems reasonable to leave 5 ml behind but to attempt to drain 20 ml.

It is generally agreed that Myodil should be drained from the basal cisterns and skull, but this can be done by putting the patient into an erect posture.

Normal appearances—Some appearances can mislead. The dorsal aspect of the vertebral bodies is relatively concave, allowing Myodil to "pool". The "pools" are connected by a narrow column which lies over the discs. This "hour glass" waisting is much less obvious when large volumes are used.

The posterior longitudinal ligament is thrown into folds during extension of the cervical spine, and thereby produces indentation of the Myodil column in lateral films.

As the Myodil column reaches the dorso-cervical junction there is usually some delay, and then the contrast medium divides, leaving a central translucence which represents the cervical cord. The lateral gutters of the spinal canal emphasise this translucency.

The root-sheaths lie in an almost truly lateral position and are normally seen. When the canal is well filled, a lateral view shows the dentate ligaments as linear translucencies. These structures may be discontinuous in cervical spondylosis in which condition they may anchor the cord and thus prevent its retreat from anterior compression.

(B) Pneumomyelography

In a beautifully illustrated paper Crandall and Hanafee (1964) discuss the value of air myelography in cervical spondylotic myelopathy. According to their technique the patient lies on his side in a 30 to 40 degrees Trendelenburg position. No lateral bending is allowed. A cisternal puncture is performed with the head in forward flexion, the needle being directed superiorly towards the deepest point of the cisterna magna. Oxygen is exchanged with cerebro-spinal fluid in increments of 10 ml. When no more fluid can be withdrawn oxygen is injected to raise the intraspinal pressure to 200–300 mm of water. Five lateral tomograms of the cervical spine are taken at 0·5 cm intervals; these obviate the need for an A.P. film which is in any case of little value since the trachea is superimposed. As an alternative standard lateral and oblique films can be used to demonstrate lateral defects.

It is necessary to carry out tomography with the patient in the head down position. The apparatus must provide for this and be fitted with shoulder slings. The method fully demonstrates both the anterior and posterior subarachnoid space, the cord, and the bony and soft tissue boundaries of the canal.

(3) Discography This consists of injecting 35 per cent Diodrast directly into the disc. It enables the radiologist to visualise the disc in a patient in whom myelography has given negative or equivocal results. The technique is described in Shapiro's book (1962).

Although it is occasionally useful in lumbar disc disease, the consensus of opinion is that discography has no useful role in the study of the cervical spine (Shapiro and Feinberg, 1964; Holt, 1964).

(4) Vertebral arteriography Direct puncture of the vertebral artery with the needle pointing towards the head permits opacification of that part of the vessel only which lies distal to the needle. It is possible by injecting downwards against the stream, to outline the whole of the artery.

Other methods include direct subclavian puncture in a retrograde ("against the flow") direction. This has disadvantages: extravasation of dye is not uncommon and it is difficult to maintain the position of the needle while the head is turned. As symptoms of vertebro-basilar insufficiency are liable to occur only when the head is turned this manoeuvre is an essential part of the examination. Also there is a real risk of pneumothorax and mediastinal haemorrhage (Sugar, 1961; Schechter, 1961; Shimidzu, 1937; Lindgren, 1950).

This review of vertebral arteriography is based upon the splendid paper by Tatelman and Sheehan (1962) which should be consulted. After considering the methods available, these authors concluded that brachial artery catheterisation as reported by Pygott and Hutton (1959) is the most suitable method. The catheter is inserted under local anaesthesia according to Seldinger's (1953) method. The catheter is advanced to a point near the origin of the vertebral artery and 20 ml of 60 per cent Renografin (Urografin) injected by hand for each exposure. Four views are taken: an A.P. of the head and neck; Towne's projection of the skull to show a semi-frontal view of the basilar artery and its intracranial branches; two views of the neck in the A.P. direction with the head turned to the right and to the left respectively.

Tatelman and Sheehan commenting on the five clinically significant complications in 220 cases, described mild thrombophlebitis of the arm, transient blindness and a hypotensive episode with mental confusion. Prompt recovery occurred with conservative management. The only serious complication occurred in a demented man who tore the pressure dressing from his arm and this led to brachial artery occlusion by a haematoma.

It is also possible to puncture the brachial artery percutaneously using a high pressure injecting technique. The aortic arch can also be reached by retrograde femoral artery catheterisation.

(5) Barium swallow This is likely to be the first examination carried out on patients with dysphagia due to osteophytosis; it should be followed by complete radiographic examination of the cervical spine.

Minimal Radiographic Examination

For the patient who has an indefinite history and no abnormal clinical signs it is probably sufficient to take only one lateral erect view of the neck.

But for the patient with a suggestive history with or without clinical signs the question remains: which of these views should be taken? Bull (1948) suggested that the minimum examination should consist of A.P., lateral and two obliques. Brain (1963) would add lateral views in flexion and extension, suggests the use of the "off lateral" zygapophyseal joint views, and says that the A.P. lateral flexion films are sometimes helpful.

The following routine is suggested:

(1) Antero-posterior view with moving jaw (2) Flexion } laterals (3) Extension } laterals	If these are normal the "neutral" film is unlikely to show a significant postural change.
(4 and 5) Both obliques	These two will give two views of the apophyseal joints—if they are normal, one or two clear spaces will be seen with no osteophytes.

If these are all normal I do not believe that many plain film mistakes will occur. We have now two possibilities which require further investigation:

(1) *Plain films normal but symptoms not explained:* This is an indication for myelography.

(2) *Plain films abnormal:* The abnormalities must be further analysed with special plain views and/or tomography and/or myelography and/or vertebral arteriography.

Normal Appearances

Structure. The accompanying normal radiographs illustrate the appearances in a healthy 40-year-old male. The following points should be borne in mind when examining the films:

In the A.P. view the neck should be held straight. The vertical bodies should be clearly defined and symmetrical. There should be no irregularity, sclerosis or erosion of the neuro-central joints, which are projected over the lateral limits of the discs. The possibilities of congenital variation must be borne in mind because it is this view which shows hemivertebrae and other variants (see Figs. 5.26–31).

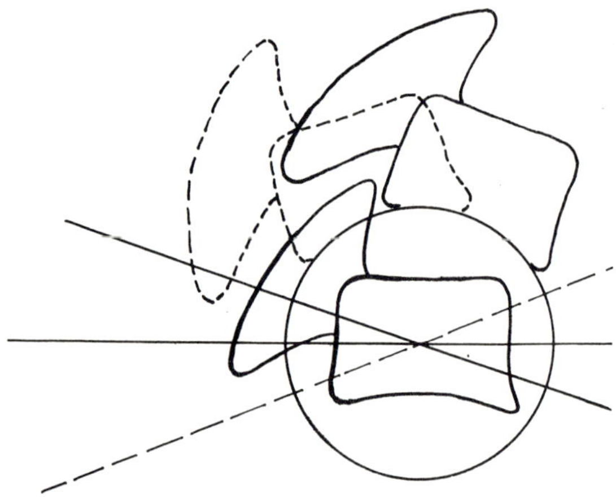

Fig. 5.5 Showing the relative movement of one vertebra on the vertebra below it in flexion (full line) and extension (dotted line)

The lateral views should next be examined. The posture of the spine is shown in two views and some impression can be gained of the relative movement between one body and another. Limitation of movement is the most common finding but in rheumatoid arthritis and in some cases of trauma there will be abnormal forward shift in flexion. For this reason it is important that a good view is gained of the atlanto-axial articulation. Although it may sound a little too elementary, it is very useful to number the vertebral bodies with a wax pencil in this and in other views. This ensures that each vertebra has been studied in turn and that the findings in lateral films can be compared with those in oblique films. The lateral films often give information as to zygapophyseal sclerosis. Again, the height and form of the bodies must be checked and especially the plate of cortical bone which is adjacent to the disc, since its disappearance is the earliest sign of pyogenic or tuberculous osteomyelitis. The spinous processes must be examined for normal appearance, erosion or fracture. It is probably advisable to look at the discs last of all since the tendency to examine these first and be preoccupied with them, may lead to the omission of a small but significant bony lesion. The oblique views are primarily designed to show the foramina and their relationship to the neuro-central and apophyseal joints. These views allow further analysis of previously noted sub-luxation and dislocation in some cases of trauma, and will be the only views which show apophyseal sub-luxation.

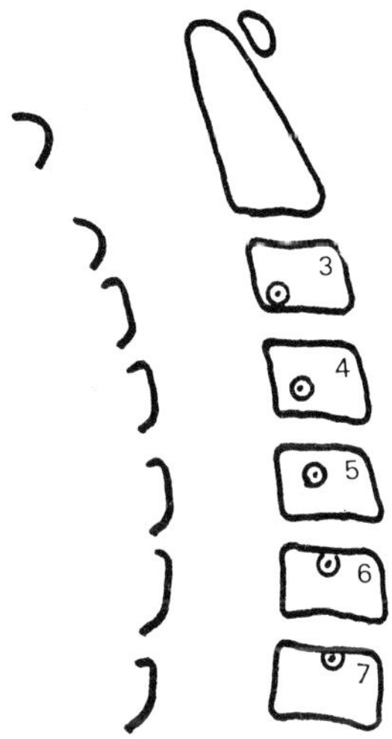

Fig. 5.6 The centres of rotation vary from one body to another and lie on a smooth curve

FLEXION AND EXTENSION MOVEMENTS IN THE CERVICAL SPINE

During flexion and extension each of the vertebrae from the axis to D1 slides forwards or backwards on the vertebra below it. The path travelled approximates to the arc of a circle centred at the body of the adjacent vertebra (Fig. 5.5.). The centre of rotation varies from one level to another (Fig. 5.6).

As a result of this motion films taken in flexion show a step like pattern along the anterior aspect of the spinal column, which is reversed in extension. The "steps" lie on a smooth curve but are not necessarily of uniform depth since not all vertebrae are equally mobile nor do they have a uniform radius of rotation. Adults have a much more even step pattern than children, in whom the greater mobility at C2–3 and C3–4 may lead to an erroneous diagnosis of subluxation (Penning, 1964). The step pattern is affected by the position of the head, which may, being flexed, affect the upper vertebrae while the lower spine is extended.

Juhl *et al.* (1962) studied flexion and extension in 116 normal subjects in order to assess angulation and displacement after cervical trauma. The neutral position showed that only 70 of 116 subjects had a convex anterior curve. In 22 it was straight, 16 had reversal of the curve while 8 had angulation as well as reversal. More frequent changes are found in the "military position", 24 of the patients presenting an angulation. (In the military position the neck is extended and the head flexed.) The authors concluded that minor variations can be found in all projections but particularly in those taken with voluntary muscle contraction. They believe that minor variations of reversal and/ or angulation of the cervical curve are not necessarily evidence of previous injury since voluntary contraction increases the incidence and extent of these changes, and that muscle contraction resulting from cervical pain is likely to be a major factor in producing alterations in the curve. They found much more uniformity in the alignment of vertebral bodies in hyperextension than in any of the other projections. Angulations presenting in the neutral or flexed positions consistently disappeared in hyperexten-

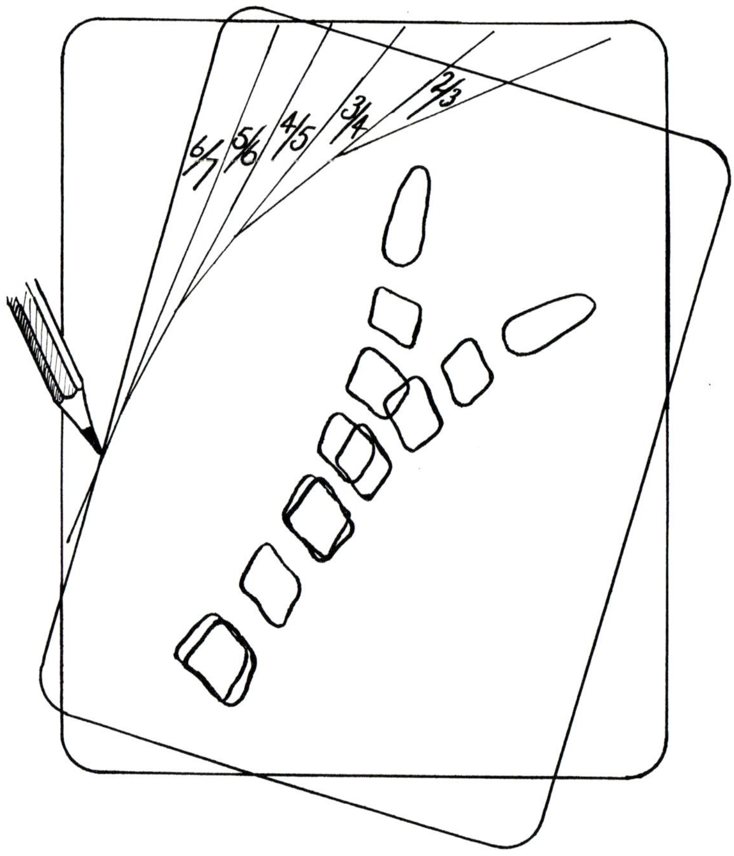

Fig. 5.7 In this method of measuring angulation the extension film is traced on to a clear film (here shown tilted). As each traced body is applied to the film taken in flexion, a line is drawn along the edge of the traced film on to flexion film

sion; this suggests that angulation of the curve in hyperextension is of more significance than in any other view (Fig. 5.34).

In their opinion, there may be little correlation between severity of injury, symptoms and radiological change. Hadley (1944) believed that a minor degree of injury may result in straightening of the lordosis while forward angulation indicates bilateral subluxation between the second and third segment in normal children. This is accompanied by a forward offset of C2 on C3 of up to 2–3 mm.

The extreme amplitude of movement between adjacent vertebrae can be measured by the method of Niemyer and Penning (1963). These authors give the normal values shown in Table 5.1.

These measurements were arrived at in this way: the extension film was traced and the tracing applied to the film taken in flexion. The method is best appreciated diagrammatically (Fig. 5.7). Normal movements of bodies depend upon the integrity of the zygapophyseal joints.

TABLE 5.1 *Average and maximum and minimum range of flexion-extension amplitude in young adults (degrees)*

	Average	*Range*
C2–3	12½	8–16
C3–4	18	13–26
C4–5	20	15–29
C5–6	21½	16–29
C6–7	15½	12–25
C7–D1	10	8–12

RADIOGRAPHIC MEASUREMENTS OF THE CERVICAL SPINE

Height of Discs and Bodies

Absolute measurements here are of less use than measuring the ratio of the body to the disc. Payne (1959) gives the following values in 15 males and 15 females (Table 5.2).

As a rule of thumb, the disc is half the height of the body below it.

TABLE 5.2 *The ratio of the height of the intervertebral disc to height of the lower adjacent vertebral body from normal radiographs of 15 males and 15 females*

	C2–3/C3	*C3–4/C4*	*C4–5/C5*	*C5–6/C6*	*C6–7/C7*
Disc height as % of body height (males)	42·9	46·5	46·7	45·3	44·2
Disc height as % of body height (females)	47·9	46·7	45·5	49·2	47·4

Antero-Posterior Diameter of the Spinal Canal

This is the most useful measurement in cervical spondylosis since it is generally agreed that it is in a narrow canal that cord compression is most likely to occur.

Wolf *et al.* (1956) measured the distance from the posterior aspect of the body to the cortical line of the spinous process in 200 adults, according to the method shown (Fig. 5.8). The films were taken lateral, erect and at 6 ft distance. The results are shown

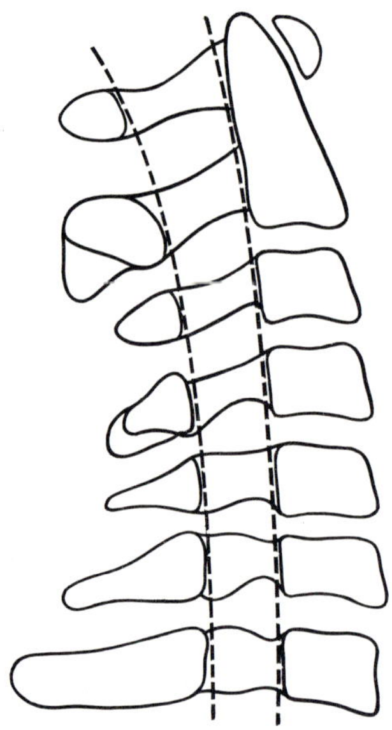

Fig. 5.8 Continuous lines are drawn along the most anterior part of the spinous processes and along the most posterior part of the vertebral bodies. The antero-posterior diameter of the spinal canal at any level is determined by the distance between the two dotted lines

in an idealised curve in Fig. 5.9. The measurements for any patient can be plotted and compared for size and gradation.

When the canal is narrowed by osteophytes, the smallest A.P. measurement is usually between a spur on the inferior posterior aspect of the vertebral body and the base of the spinous process of the vertebra below (Fig. 5.10). The body moves forward in flexion, and this diameter may be about 2 mm less in full extension. Cord compression may be expected if the sagittal diameter at any level is 10 mm or less with the head in a central position. When the minimum diameter is from 10–13 mm cord compression may or may not be present. If the measurement is 13 mm or greater it is unlikely that simple spondylotic changes are the cause of cord compression.

It is still possible that uncalcified extruded disc material might be contributing to cord compression, but it would usually only do this if the original diameter were on the small side. In a patient with signs of cord compression in whom a space-occupying lesion is suspected, adequate sagittal diameters suggest that the lesion is in the cord or meninges rather than the discs.

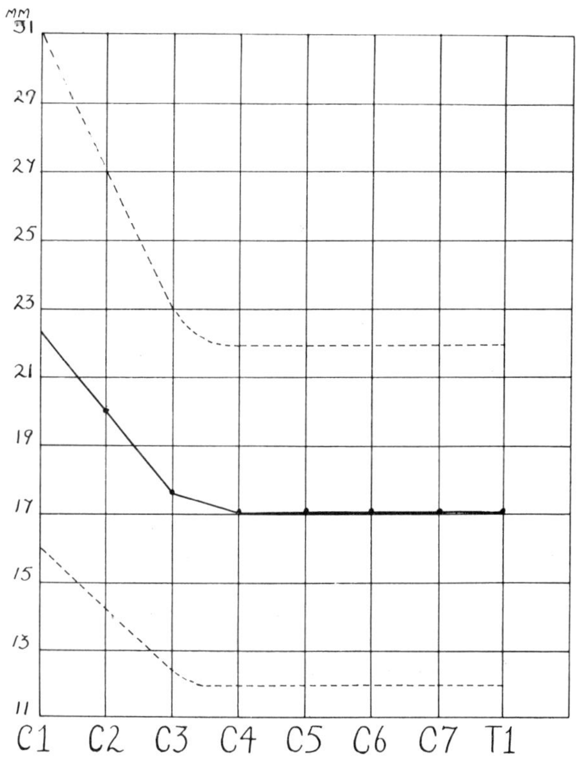

Fig. 5.9 Maximum, minimum and average measurements of the antero-posterior dimensions of the spinal canal

The spur seen in a lateral film may not be in the midline, therefore a measurement taken from it cannot represent a truly sagittal diameter. Myelography may demonstrate a laterally placed projection obliterating the root pouch. Nevertheless, the measurement is still of value, since it leads the examiner to investigate further with myelography. Crandall and Hanafee (1964) give the following values:

Canal	12–22 mm with average 17 mm from C3–4/C6–7.
Cord average	9·5 mm at C3–4 tapering to 8 mm at C6–7 varying ±1 mm.

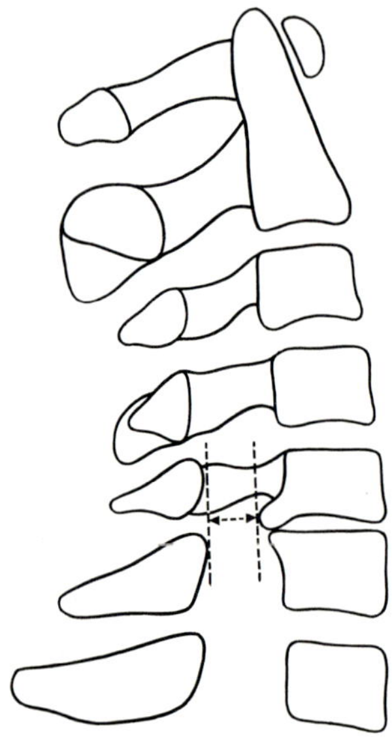

Fig. 5.10

The cord retains its relative position in the sagittal plane because it is anchored by the roots and dentate ligaments.

Payne (1959) gives the following values: in normal patients (Table 5.3), with cervical spondylosis without myelography (Table 5.4) and patients with cervical spondylosis with cervical myelography (Table 5.5).

TABLE 5.3 *The antero-posterior diameter (mm) of the normal cervical spinal canal from lateral radiographs of 85 adults*

	15 MALES		15 FEMALES	
	Mean	*Range*	*Mean*	*Range*
C1	21·5	20·0–26·0	21·6	18·0–24·0
C2	19·9	17·5–23·0	19·8	18·0–22·0
C3	18·6	14·5–22·0	17·9	16·0–20·0
C4	17·5	14·0–20·0	17·3	15·0–20·0
C5	17·8	15·0–22·0	17·1	15·0–19·0
C6	17·8	16·5–21·0	17·0	15·0–18·0
C7	17·8	16·5–20·0	16·6	14·5–18·5

TABLE 5.4 *Cervical spondylosis without myelography*

	15 MALES		15 FEMALES	
	Mean	*Range*	*Mean*	*Range*
C1	21·0	18·5–23·0	21·4	16·5–24·0
C2	18·2	16·0 20·0	18·5	15·0–21·0
C3	16·3	15·0–18·0	16·4	13·0–18·5
C4	15·4	13·5–18·0	15·3	13·0–17·5
C5	15·0	13·0–18·5	14·8	12·0–16·5
C6	14·8	13·0–18·0	14·8	12·5–16·0
C7	15·3	13·0–19·0	15·1	12·5–17·0

TABLE 5.5 *Cervical spondylosis with cervical myelography*

	15 MALES		15 FEMALES	
	Mean	*Range*	*Mean*	*Range*
C1	20·7	16·0–25·5	20·5	17·0–24·0
C2	18·1	15·0–21·5	17·4	15·0–21·0
C3	16·1	12·5–21·0	15·0	13·0–18·0
C4	14·5	12·0–18·0	14·4	12·0 18·0
C5	14·4	12·0–17·0	14·1	12·5–17·0
C6	14·0	11·0–17·0	14·1	11·5–17·0
C7	14·3	11·0–17·0	14·6	13·0–16·0

Atlanto-Axial Articulation

The maximum distance between the posterior border of the anterior arch of the atlas and the odontoid process in health has been variously estimated. Conlon *et al.* (1966) regarded 2·5 mm and 3 mm as being the upper normal limit for females and males respectively. Tishler *et al.* (1965) regarded the upper limit at 5 mm in all patients including children in whom the distance is usually wider than in adults. They describe the prevalence of dislocation of the atlas in mongolism illustrated by 4 out of 18 mongols in whom this interval exceeds 5 mm.

Dugan *et al.* (1962), describing increased motility of the atlanto-axial joint as a cause of occipital neuralgia in adolescents and young adults, give 2 mm as the usual distance between the peg and the anterior arch of the atlas and state that neurological signs are likely if the odontoid moves more than 3 mm "back and forth".

The possibility of atlanto-axial dislocation is well recognised. It is worth mentioning that in arthritis this distance might be reduced by erosion (Fig. 5.11).

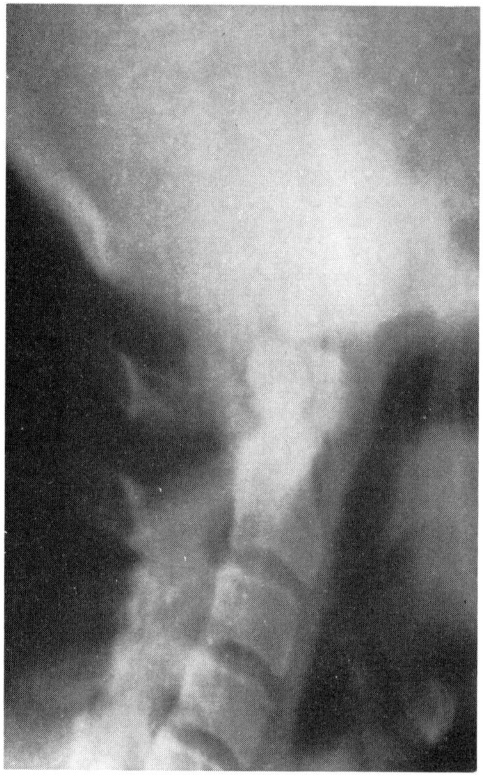

Fig. 5.11 Tomograph to show erosion, sclerosis and narrowing of the atlanto-axial joint in ankylosing spondylitis

RADIOLOGICAL SIGNS OF CERVICAL SPONDYLOSIS

Plain Film Changes

Discs When the nucleus pulposus suddenly herniates into the spinal canal or into a foramen, there are usually no abnormalities in the static films. There might be alterations in the posture of the cervical spine with limitation of movement but, as already explained, such changes are common in health and are not alone sufficiently reliable for diagnosis.

The affected disc is sometimes narrow; if it is the only narrow disc this finding is significant especially if there is a marked postural change. If there are several narrow discs, precise localisation is impossible without myelography.

Disc narrowing is an almost constant feature of cervical spondylosis and is primarily due to dehydration of the nucleus pulposus, followed by disc degeneration. The disc becomes more or less squeezed out between the vertebral margins, especially anteriorly, and this protrusion is followed by the formation of osteophytes. These lesions are commonest at the level C5–6 and almost as common at C6–7. When they are multiple, the C5–6 disc is almost always diseased. Sometimes, especially in the early stages, only one disc is involved and this is likely to be one of these two. Narrowing of the upper discs by themselves is unlikely to be due to spondylosis alone.

The height of the discs can be seen in the lateral films. The full extent of their protrusion may not be seen in plain films since the soft tissue may be in advance of the

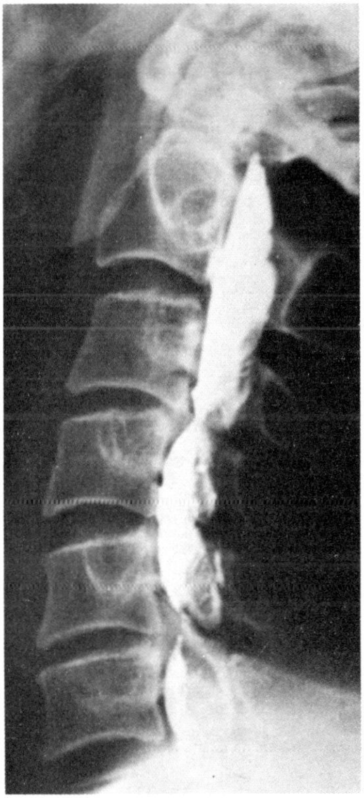

Fig. 5.12 Cervical spondylosis with disc protrusion at C3–4 and 5–6 with little bony change

accompanying osteophytes (Fig. 5.12); also acute herniation of the nucleus may occur during this degenerative process. Nevertheless it would be difficult to sustain the diagnosis of spondylotic myelopathy without well defined posterior osteophytes.

Bodies When the disc is narrowed in spondylosis the adjacent vertebral bodies are either normal, which is unusual, or show varying degrees of sclerosis and osteophytosis. Sclerosis is seen in the cortical bone which is immediately related to the disc.

Patchy sclerosis elsewhere in the body is due to some other cause such as secondary carcinoma, fluorosis or Paget's disease. The cortical bone is not eroded in spondylosis; erosion with disc narrowing suggests an inflammatory lesion such as rheumatoid arthritis or tuberculosis. Osteophytosis may occur at any or all points on the periphery of the intervertebral disc.

Anterior osteophytes buttress the bodies against movement, like outriggers in a

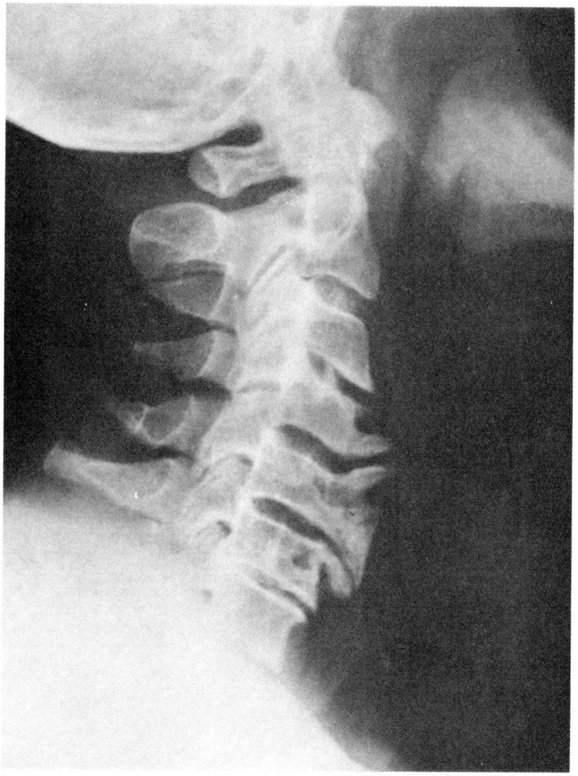

Fig. 5.13 Gross osteophytosis causing locking of neck. The discs are relatively well preserved

canoe; sometimes they are so large as to alter completely the shape of the bodies (Fig. 5.13). Osteophytes increase the load-bearing area in proportion to the square of their radius, so that in this way as by limiting movement they have a protective and compensatory function. Occasionally anterior osteophytes impinge upon the neighbouring structures causing hoarseness and dysphagia. These symptoms may be precipitated by trauma. Anterior osteophytes occasionally fuse.

Posterior osteophytes tend to be smaller, but since they occupy the spinal canal and are often accompanied by a more extensive protrusion of soft tissue, they are much more important clinically. They cannot be precisely located on plain films. If they seem likely to be contributing to the clinical picture, lateral tomography or myelography is necessary to show their position. The compressive effect of osteophytes

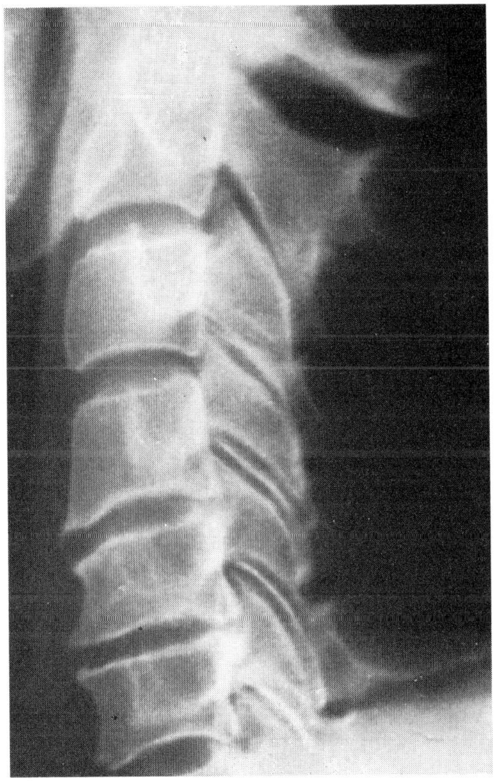

Fig. 5.14 Even moderate posterior osteophytosis seen here at C4–5, C5–6, may have a profound effect in a congenitally small canal. Here the sagittal diameter at C5–6 is only 10 mm (by courtesy of Dr. David Sutton)

depends largely upon the original diameter of the spinal canal (Fig. 5.14). If the clinical X-ray shows a sagittal diameter of 13 mm or more it is unlikely that simple spondylotic changes, including soft tissue protrusion, are the sole cause of cord compression.

A postero-lateral osteophyte is unlikely to compress the cord but may compress the nerve root by encroaching upon the foramen. These osteophytes are best seen in the oblique views and correspond to degenerative changes in the neurocentral joints.

Since these joints also occupy the lateral aspect of the inter-body articulation, they can also be seen in the antero-posterior views. The direction of neurocentral osteophytes varies with the plane of the joint surfaces—postero-laterally both are more or less horizontal; laterally they have an upward and outward direction and may compress the vertebral artery. Thus these osteophytes follow the general rule: that their original direction is in the plane of the joint from which they arise.

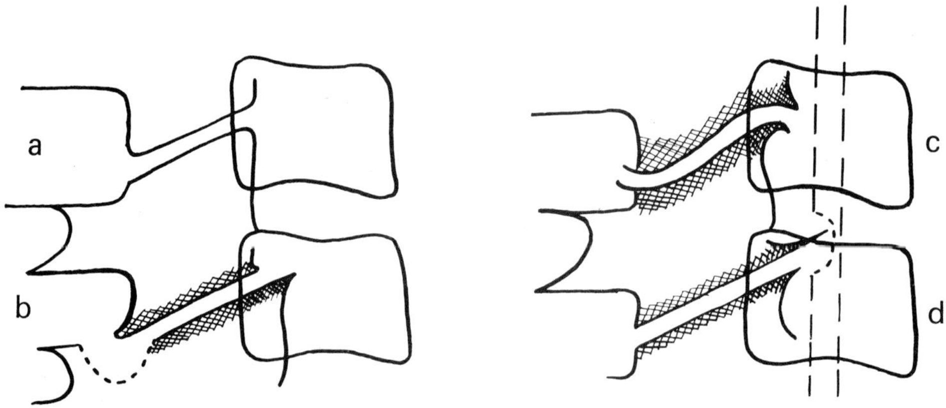

Fig. 5.15 Spondylotic changes in the zygapophyseal joint (schematic)

a. Normal.
b. Posterior slipping of the superior facet with erosion of the lamina.
c. Locking of the zygapophyseal joint by anterior and posterior "hooking" of osteophytes. Note that the vertebral artery (interrupted line is not at risk).
d. The anterior osteophyte threatens the vertebral artery.

Zygapophyseal joints Degenerative changes in these joints, called osteoarthrosis by some and osteoarthritis by others, are an integral feature of spondylosis. The upper rather than the lower joints are most commonly affected. The joints, which are synovial, show the classical changes of osteoarthritis: narrowing of cartilage, sclerosis of bony margins and osteophytosis. When these changes are severe they can be seen in the A.P. view (Fig. 5.28). For earlier signs and for detailed assessment, other views are required (see "Radiography" above).

As a result of spondylosis the superior articular surfaces tend to slip backwards and may erode the laminae below (Fig. 5.15b). Sometimes the slipping movement is prevented by an upward pointing osteophyte (Fig. 5.15c) arising from either the lamina or transverse process (Kovacs, 1955). Anterio-medial osteophytes may abut against the pedicle and turn horizontally then downwards, interlocking and preventing backward subluxation (Fig. 5.15c). Projections of this sort do not reach the vertebral artery, but do jeopardise the spinal root by narrowing the foramen (Fig. 5.16).

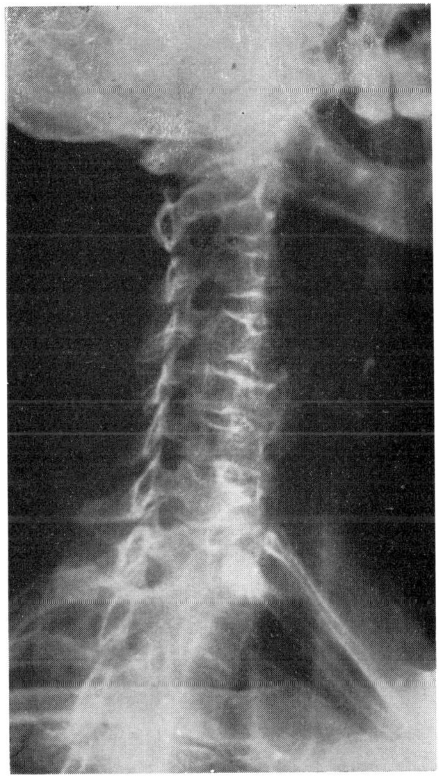

Fig. 5.16 Gross zygapophyseal joint changes at C4–5 and C5–6. The distribution is characteristic in the upper zygapophyseal joint changes and lower disc changes but note the effect on the foramen C4–5 which is encroached upon by osteophytes from the zygapophyseal joint and the neurocentral joint. All the neurocentral joints below this are involved

More laterally placed anterior osteophytes tend to grow anteriorly so as to threaten the vertebral artery (Fig. 5.15d). Whether or not they reach the artery depends partly upon the original relationship of the joint and vessel—this varies in different people.

Zygapophyseal subluxation also threatens the artery. Kovacs has published films taken during an attack of headache and remission showing respectively subluxation and reduction. The threat by zygapophyseal osteophytes is shown in Figure 5.17.

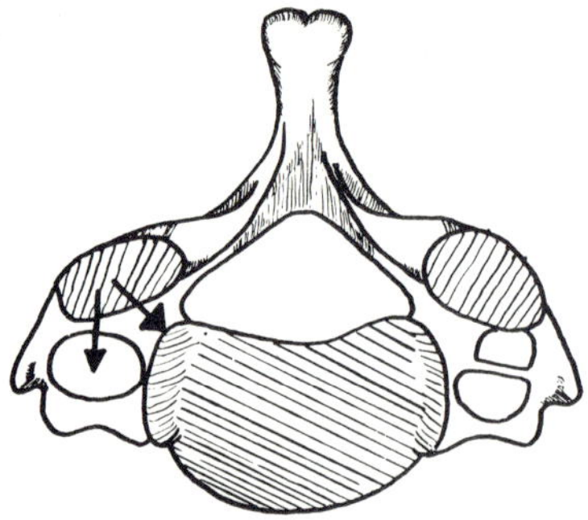

Fig. 5.17 Zygapophyseal osteophytosis may develop antero-medially compressing the canal, or anteriorly compressing the artery, or both may occur; note direction of arrows from the articular facet. Anterior projection is best seen in the off lateral view film (see Fig. 5.3b)

Foramina Zygapophyseal and neurocentral osteophytes may encroach upon the foramina together. Since zygapophyseal changes occur mainly in the upper, and neurocentral changes mainly in the lower cervical spine, their combined encroachment is first seen in the mid cervical region (Fig. 5.16). Encroachment of this kind is not usually symmetrical owing to the different relative position of the two joints (Fig. 5.18).

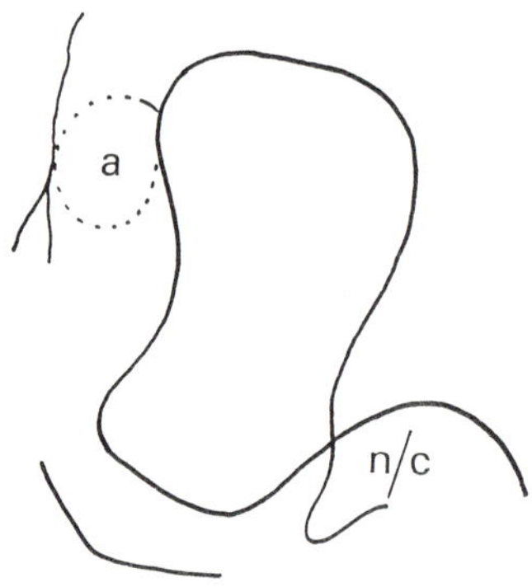

Fig. 5.18 Relative positions of zygapophyseal joint (a) and neurocentral (n/c) in the periphery of the foramina (schematic)

Vertebral arteries The vertebral arteries may be compressed by lateral neurocentral osteophytes (Fig. 5.19), by zygapophyseal osteophytes, and by the inferior articular facet during posterior subluxation. Even in combination these effects do not usually give rise to symptoms unless the artery is already atheromatous. And even so, the symptoms of gross narrowing often only occur when the head is turned to the affected side (Tatelman and Sheehan, 1962). The situation is not entirely one-sided, since bone in contact with the artery tends to be eroded. Presumably the transient compression caused by turning the head does not last long enough for this erosion to take place. Also, soft tissue protrusions, being more resistant to erosion, may play an important part (note middle arrow in Fig. 5.19).

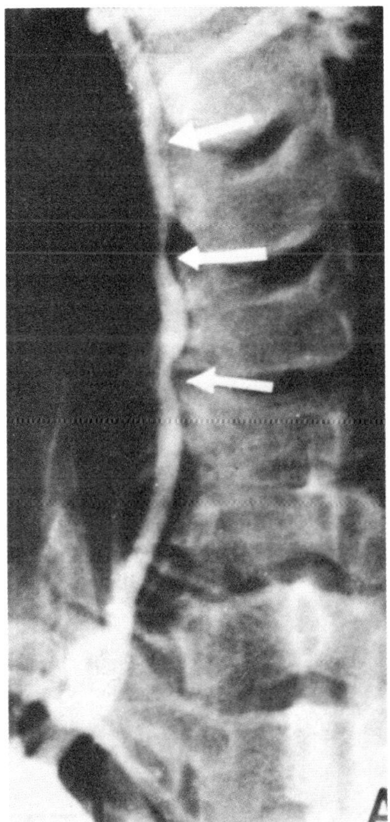

Fig. 5.19 Narrowing and kinking of the vertebral artery by lateral disc protrusion. The middle arrow shows a mainly soft tissue impression while the lower arrow shows a projection which is almost entirely due to osteophytes (by courtesy of Dr. John Meyer)

Kinking of the vertebral artery also causes erosion of bone. The defect has a sclerotic margin; myelography is normal and the diagnosis made by arteriography. Forwards subluxation of the cervical spine may also be accompanied by arterial erosion of the anterior surface of the superior facet.

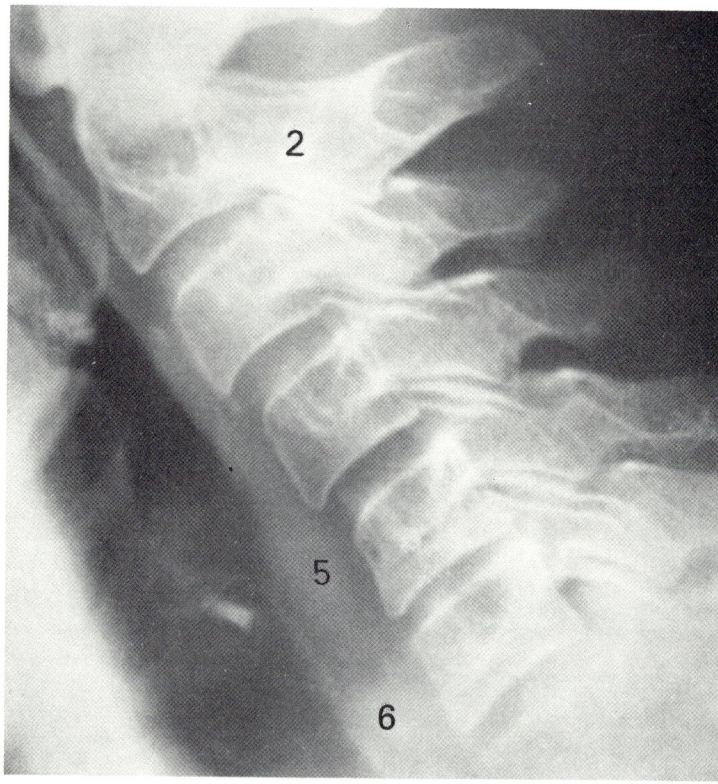

Fig. 5.20 Narrowing of the disc with mild posterior osteophytosis inhibiting movement in forward flexion at C5–6. Note also the absence of movement of C2 on C3 associated with high zygapophyseal sclerosis

Abnormality of movement Spondylotic changes inhibit movement between one vertebra and another (Fig. 5.20). There may be some subluxation either forward or backwards, but this is more likely to be static than dynamic. Increased movement, especially in flexion, occurs in joints which are normal or not severely affected immediately above those which are immobilised (Fig. 5.21). This disproportionate movement is compensatory. As already described, movement is inhibited by osteophytosis of the bodies and by osteophytosis in the zygapophyseal joints. Movement of bodies is limited in two ways; protrusion of the disc with accompanying osteophytosis increases the radius of rotation (the outrigger effect) and therefore increases stability.

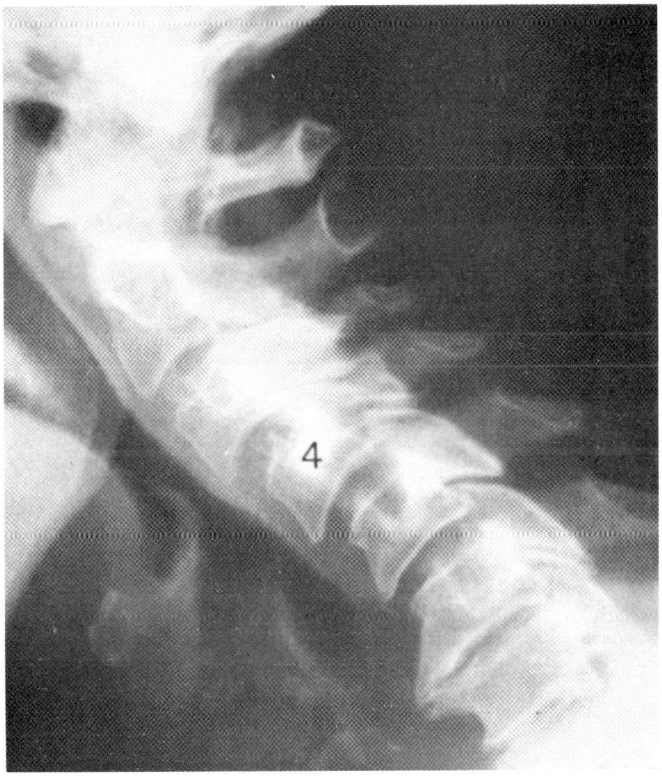

Fig. 5.21 Exaggerated forward movement of C4 on C5 associated with marked disc lesions at C6–7 (by courtesy of Dr. David Sutton)

Also the disc is less elastic and narrower than normal, so that it is less able to "give" with movement. When the relative motion of two or more bodies is restricted by disease, the increased movement of normal segments is likely to precipitate spondylosis even sooner than might be expected. In the same way lateral flexion of the cervical spine is also inhibited.

MYELOGRAPHIC SIGNS OF CERVICAL SPONDYLOSIS

Myelography is useful:

(1) to exclude an operable lesion when the clinical and laboratory findings are inconclusive and when the working diagnosis is degenerative disease.
(2) to confirm an intra-spinal lesion especially in patients with extensive spondylosis and definite clinical findings.
(3) to establish the nature and extent of a known lesion.
(4) to exclude multiple lesions.
(5) to determine the cause of symptoms after laminectomy.

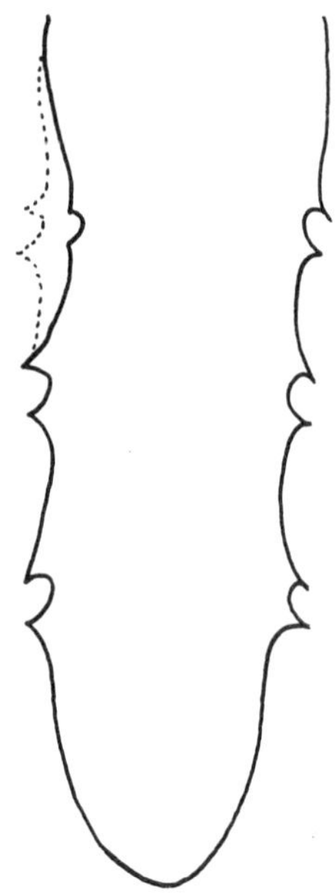

Fig. 5.22 Displacement of the Myodil column without obliteration of the root sheath

Myelographic signs in cervical spondylosis

Myelography demonstrates both bony and soft tissue encroachment upon the subarachnoid space, and hence the spinal cord. It also shows whether the nerve root sheaths are filled or not. Positive contrast myelography is most commonly used in this country, and the following description applied to this method. Cervical spondylosis produces central and lateral filling defects. There may be one or several central defects, one or several lateral defects, or the films may show a combination of these. All these defects are caused by deformity of the dura, and can therefore be classed as extra-dural filling defects. If they exceed the bony protrusions, they must include soft tissues. If they are not accompanied by bony protrusions, they are due only to soft tissue lesions—and these include disc or nucleus pulposus (or both) and may be acute or chronic, depending upon the clinical picture.

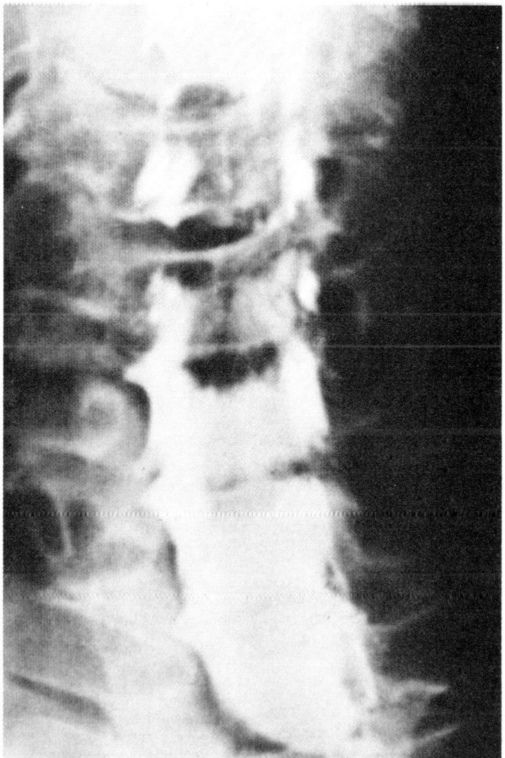

Fig. 5.23 Multiple transverse bars simulating intramedullary neoplasm. The film also illustrates various degrees of root sheath obliteration. Note complete obliteration at the 2nd and 3rd interspace down on the left of the print and at the 2nd, 3rd and 4th interspace on the right

The simplest lateral defect is medial displacement of the Myodil column without deformity of the nerve root sheath (Fig. 5.22). More commonly the sheath is obliterated and usually accompanied by a semicircular defect of the column (Fig. 5.23).

When lateral soft tissue protrusion occurs in spondylosis the defect in the Myodil column extends a little more medially than the "spurring" seen to arise from the neurocentral joint in the plain films. Lateral defects may also be large and irregular and extend towards the midline. They are often best seen at the shallow edge of the Myodil pool.

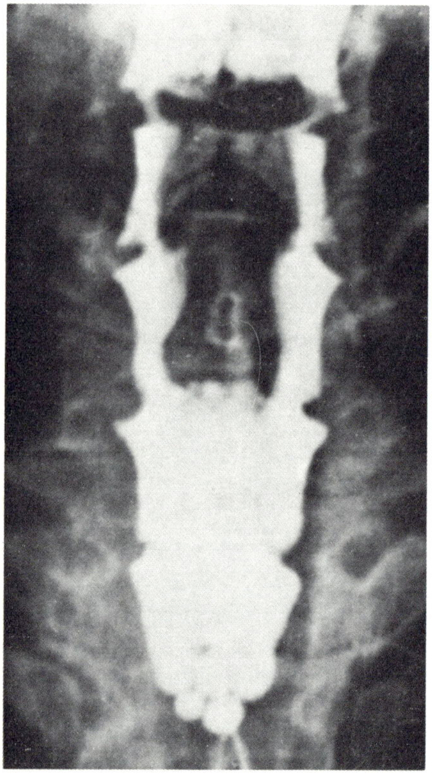

Fig. 5.24a Central filling defect due to posteriorly protruded discs. Note normal filling of the root sheaths

Posterior defects are exaggerated by extension of the neck because of the "kinking" of the posterior longitudinal ligament. They may extend across the whole width of the disc (hence they are called transverse bars, Figs. 5.23 and 5.24a), or may stop short on one side or both. Since their effect is to compress the cord, they are responsible for apparent widening of it and may thus simulate an intramedullary tumour in the A.P. view. Gliomata usually cause more widening over a much longer distance than spondylosis but confusion can occasionally arise with extensive spondylosis. Fortunately the lateral view provides the solution, since intramedullary lesions also increase the sagittal diameter of the cord while spondylosis shows characteristic narrowings opposite to the discs (Fig. 5.24b).

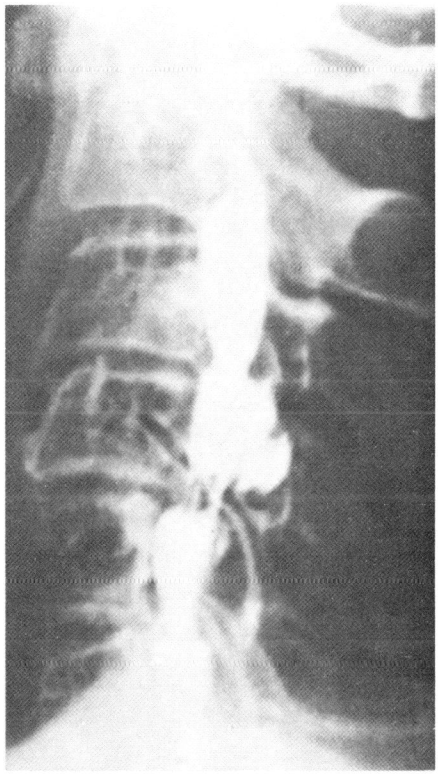

Fig. 5.24b The lateral projection shows the posterior protrusions which are not accompanied by gross osteophytosis

Abnormal findings in a myelogram may be only partly due to spondylosis, which is a common condition. The observer must be on the look-out for co-existing lesions which might be responsible for the patient's symptoms and signs.

When the patient is tilted into the head down position the Myodil column may be held in the cervical region for several minutes by a transverse bar. It sometimes trickles slowly past one or both sides when it is held up in the centre.

McRae (1956) likens a stream of Myodil to water flowing over a dam and thus explains the narrowing of the column as it flows over a transverse bar. This seems specious. It is obvious that water flowing out over a dam (or out of a tumbler) proceeds in an ever narrowing stream, but this is a function of acceleration and surface tension. It is hard to imagine how these conditions apply to a slow moving column of Myodil in the cerebro-spinal fluid. In fact, if the velocity of the column is uniform, then on this analogy the stream must widen since its depth is suddenly decreased. The narrowing of the column is more likely to be due to bilateral indentation of the dura or to "pooling" of the stream referred to above. In multiple protrusions Myodil tends to lie in the gutters leaving a central deformity. It seems likely that detailed dynamic conclusions cannot be drawn from the very slow moving stream. McRae also warns against misinterpreting peculiar impressions in patients with shallow lateral gutters (but these impressions alternate with root sheaths).

INCIDENCE AND SIGNIFICANCE OF THE RADIOLOGICAL SIGNS OF CERVICAL SPONDYLOSIS

The available information on the correlation of radiological and clinical abnormalities is of two kinds. Population studies have been carried out by Lawrence *et al.* (1963) and their co-workers to determine the incidence of osteoarthritis. In the course of their studies they have distinguished patients who have rheumatoid arthritis, and have shown that a considerable proportion of their subjects have both rheumatoid arthritis and osteoarthritis. Although in general they have shown a good correlation between peripheral osteoarthritis and radiological changes, the correlation in the cervical spine was marginal, at least as far as zygapophyseal arthrosis is concerned. The methods and results of this work are reproduced here in some detail.

Another way of approaching the problem is to examine groups of patients who are attending hospital with and without clinical evidence of cervical spondylosis. Two examples of this kind of study are dealt with. There are really two problems: first, what is the clinical significance of radiological spondylosis occurring as a chance finding? To which the answer seems to be, very little; secondly, what is the significance of radiological signs in patients who are being deliberately investigated because of clinical signs and/or symptoms? The answer to this question seems to be that on the whole the radiological findings are very helpful.

In the general population

The radiological survey carried out by Lawrence *et al.* (1963) in Leigh, Lancashire and Wensleydale, Yorkshire, included a lateral view of the cervical spine in which osteoarthritis of the zygapophyseal joints and disc degeneration were separately graded.

In order to distinguish co-existing rheumatoid arthritis in zygapophyseal arthrosis the population was divided as follows:

(1) Rheumatoid (R.A.) = Probable or definite R.A. as defined by the American Rheumatism Association's criteria.

(2) Intermediate (I.R.A.) = Not in Group 1 but having clinically definite R.A., those with past history of polyarthritis or with radiological evidence of the disease or a positive sheep-cell agglutination test.

(3) Non R.A.

Table 5.6 shows the distribution of patients in these three categories and the percentage for each grade who complained of pain.

TABLE 5.6 *Grading of zygapophyseal arthrosis with percentage of patients in each group with pain*

	No. X-rayed	*Grade 0–1*	*% c/o pain*	*Grade 2*	*% c/o pain*	*Grade 3–4*	*% c/o pain*
Non R.A.	895	812	37·1	67	38·3	16	68·7
Male:							
I.R.A.	173	144	52·1	22	45·5	7	28·6
R.A.	26	21	42·9	3	66·7	2	100
Female:							
Non R.A.	892	825	39·6	58	39·7	9	55·5
I.R.A.	222	188	64·4	22	81·8	12	66·7
R.A.	75	47	57·9	14	85·7	4	75·0

In radiologically severe arthrosis the complaint rate was only double that of the patients with normal or doubtful radiological changes. Pain was limited to the neck in some and to the shoulders in others but was generally in the neck-shoulder-brachial distribution. It is clear from the tables that a large proportion of the population complained of pain in the cervico-brachial regions. Lawrence *et al.* (1966) concluded that after standardisation of the adult population for age and sex by the unweighted mean the prevalence of osteoarthritis (with exclusion of minimal disease) was 19 per cent in males and 22 per cent in females. After comparing several joints as well as the cervical and lumbar spine the authors concluded that the non-rheumatoid group showed a significant correlation between X-ray changes of osteoarthritis and the frequency of symptoms with corresponding distribution. This was present in all joints except those of the lumbar spine and was only marginal in the cervical zygapophyseal joints.

Results in patients aged 55 and over:

Sex	*Total X-rayed*	*No disc lesion*	*Per cent with disc lesion*
Males	279	46	83·5
Females	368	71	80·7

There is a steady increase in both the prevalence and severity of disc degeneration with age, and although incidence is the same in both men and women, women tend to be less severely affected than men. In both sexes some degree of cervical disc degeneration is present in about 80 per cent of all persons over the age of 55, and it is probably

TABLE 5.7 *Prevalence of radiological evidence of disc degeneration in the cervical spine in combined Leigh and Wensleydale populations*

Age	*Total X-rayed*	*No disc degeneration*	*% of total X-rayed*	*Grades 1–4 in 4 or more discs % of total X-rayed*
MALES:				
15–24	165	155	94	0
25–34	176	147	84	0
35–44	183	114	62	0
45–54	233	76	33	2
55–64	139	35	25	12
65–74	93	8	9	19
75+	47	3	7	23
FEMALES:				
15–24	170	162	95	0
25–34	172	154	89	0
35–44	213	156	73	0
45–54	224	88	35	3
55–64	174	39	22	18
65–74	137	21	15	13
75+	57	11	2	12

true to say that a large majority of patients from other areas who are over the age of 55 will present radiological evidence of disc degeneration. Lawrence *et al.* (1963) have also compared X-ray changes of disc degeneration with symptoms in the corresponding areas for deep pain in joints of those with disc degeneration of grade 3 and 4. In just over half there was no history of pain. Nevertheless there was a significant relationship between cervical disc degeneration and neck-shoulder-brachial pain. The significance was more striking up to the age of 45, and indeed in males the association was only definite in this younger age group. Unlike lumbar disc degeneration, cervical disc degeneration is little or not at all affected by occupation.

One must question the scientific value of such elegant statistics when they are applied to what appears to be such inadequate and misleading primary evidence as is represented by a single lateral film of the cervical spine taken under poor radiographic conditions.

In hospital populations

Clinical correlation Pallis *et al.* (1954) studied 50 non-neurological patients in hospital in order to study the significance of radiographic findings in the cervical spine. They took A.P., lateral and both oblique views and classified the degree of canal narrowing and of foraminal narrowing. Posterior osteophytosis was graded as moderate or severe at the most severely affected site; subluxation was assessed according to the loss of alignment of the posterior margins of adjacent bodies as moderate or severe. Alterations of the cervical lordosis was regarded as moderate if there was straightening at any level, and severe where there was actual kyphosis.

The following composite assessment of canal narrowing was made:

(A) Severe posterior osteophytosis.
(B) Moderate posterior osteophytosis and subluxation.
(C) Moderate posterior osteophytosis and kyphosis.
(D) Kyphosis and subluxation.

Canal narrowing was regarded as being moderate where there was:

(A) Moderate posterior osteophytosis.
(B) Slight posterior osteophytosis and kyphosis.
(C) Slight posterior osteophytosis and subluxation.
(D) Severe subluxation.

Narrowing of discs was found to be striking in some cases but this was not assessed since narrowing is not necessarily accompanied by protrusion as shown myelographically.

Foraminal narrowing was graded none, slight, moderate and severe. It was found that the neurocentral joints were the commonest cause of foraminal narrowing, that zygapophyseal joint changes did not commonly cause narrowing and that the foraminal narrowing was not affected by adjacent disc narrowing.

As a result of clinical examination patients were divided into four groups:

In group 1 (16 patients) no clinical abnormality was seen of neck or nervous system.

In group 2 (four patients) the neck was clinically abnormal but the C.N.S. was normal.

In group 3 (16 patients) there were symptoms in the nervous system.

In group 4 (14 patients) there were signs of cord or root lesion.

All the patients with abnormal signs in the neck had X-ray abnormalities, but quite which were responsible did not emerge. Nearly half the patients with radiological spondylosis had clinical signs in the neck. Disc narrowing was present in 43 patients, having the following characteristic distribution:

2–3 (1) 3–4 (5) 4–5 (7) 5–6 (24) 6–7 (20) 7–1 (5)

Kyphosis was not taken into account in assessing canal or foraminal narrowing.

38 patients were regarded as having moderate (23) or severe (15) canal narrowing.
36 patients had moderate (30) or severe (6) foraminal narrowing.

The correlation was as follows:

	Per cent
Cord signs and no canal narrowing	0
Cord signs in patients with canal narrowing	58
Overall canal narrowing	78
Canal narrowing in patients with cord signs	100
Root lesions without foraminal narrowing	6

	Per cent
Root lesions in patients with foraminal narrowing	39
Overall foraminal narrowing	72
Narrow foramina in patients with root lesions	82

These findings have been dealt with in some detail because they show that careful radiography and radiological observation based on combination of signs rather than individual radiographic signs can lead to an extremely close correlation between the clinical picture and the radiological picture.

McRae (1960) studied 240 patients with and without symptoms relating to the cervical spine or to the cervical spinal cord. He found marked disc thinning, osteophyte formation at C5–6 and/or C6–7 level in more than 50 per cent of the cervical spine in patients over 40 years of age (see Table 5.8).

TABLE 5.8 *Correlation of cervical disc disease with symptoms*

	30–39 symptoms		*40–49 symptoms*		*50–59 symptoms*		*60–over symptoms*	
	+	−	+	−	+	−	+	−
No. of patients	10	48	37	54	28	22	15	26
% normal Roentgenograms C2–T1	60	25	22	28	7	13	0	0
% thin disc and posterior osteophytes at same level	10	13	45	31	53	33	60	85

Osteoarthritis of the zygapophyseal joints was almost as common as disc disease but the site of the incidence differed in that the upper zygapophyseal joints are affected rather than the lower. McRae draws the following conclusion from his studies. For the radiological changes to be significant in patients with spondylosis and clinical neurological disease, the neurological level must correspond closely to the level of radiographic abnormality. The presence of degenerative disease does not exclude other lesions. Cervical roots can remain healthy in constricted foramina if there is no extruded disc tissue and if the meninges remain pliable. Plain films show no evidence of recent lesions; a final and complete radiological opinion can be given only after myelography.

CONGENITAL ABNORMALITIES

Anomalies of the cervical spine are relatively common in clinical radiology, and are important in several ways. They may themselves cause neurological disturbance, especially in the second or third decade or they may re-inforce the effect of trauma or inflammation.

They also predispose to early spondylosis (Fig. 5.25). It is seldom easy and sometimes impossible to separate what is congenital and what is acquired. Thus Still's disease may cause fusion of the vertebral bodies in early life and produce a picture which is indistinguishable from the Klippel-Feil syndrome. Some of these distinctions

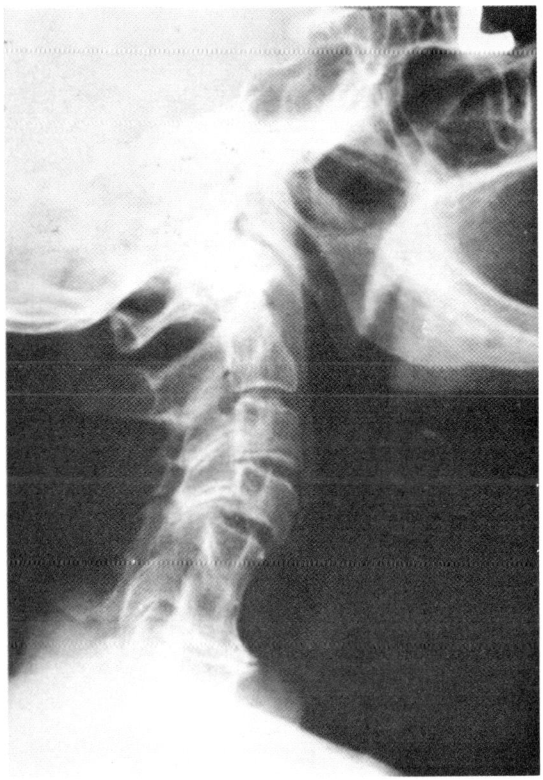

Fig. 5.25 The Klippel-Feil abnormality may predispose to cervical spondylosis. Note the subluxation and zygapophyseal arthrosis above the conjoined vertebrae and gross disc narrowing and osteophytosis below

are more academic than practical but the recognition of the congenital factor in combined disease depends upon the knowledge of possible anomalies. Agenesis and hypoplasia—these defects may occur anywhere in the cervical spine but are more common at the atlanto-occipital and cervico-dorsal junction. For example the arch of the atlas may be completely absent without trouble to the patient, but symptoms may arise when the patient acquires another disease such as rheumatoid arthritis.

A deficiency in one element may be compensated for in others. If half of a vertebra is absent or rudimentary the lateral masses above and below may enlarge and articulate together (Fig. 5.26). If the centrum is insufficiently calcified, the epiphyseal plates grow to make up the height of the body. Non-union of the secondary ossification centres in the tips of the articular processes may lead to formation of an extra zygapophyseal joint which is liable to show degenerative changes. The ossicle may articulate separately, and may impinge upon the neural arch below. This may be mistaken for a

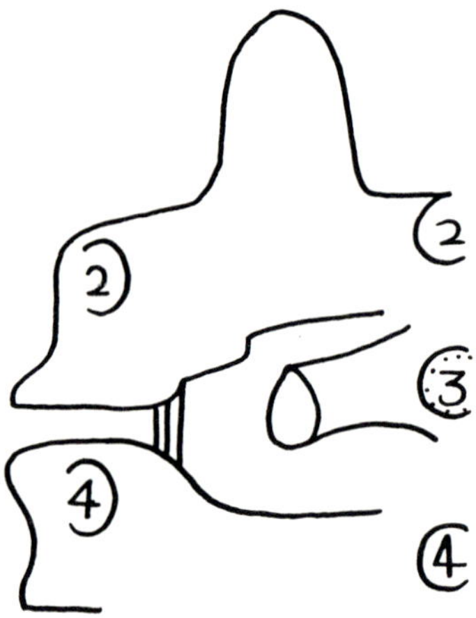

Fig. 5.26

fracture. A persistent secondary centre for the spinous process should not be confused with a fracture, nor should the ossicle frequently seen in the nuchal ligament. (It should be noted that shoveller's fracture occurs at the base of a spinous process.)

A vertebra may be separated into two halves—the so-called butterfly vertebra (Fig. 5.27).

There may be one or more hemi-vertebrae. The effect of one may be counterbalanced by another on the opposite side at a lower level (Fig. 5.23) or the effect may be enhanced by another half on the same side (Fig. 5.29).

The odontoid process is subject to various disturbances leading to increased amplitude of movement. These include absence of the odontoid, separate ossification of its tip, and non-union. These abnormalities can lead to cord compression after trauma. Absence of the odontoid is very rare. McRae (1960) noted that the Montreal Neurological Institute had no proven case. Its diagnosis requires very careful plain radiography and tomography. Separation of the odontoid may be accompanied by forward or backward dislocation which is either recurrent or chronically progressive (Fig. 5.4). Spontaneous symptoms may occur. Chronic atlanto-axial dislocation in which there is no history of injury is probably congenital in origin and often isolated. When the atlas is dislocated directly forward the odontoid presses against the medulla

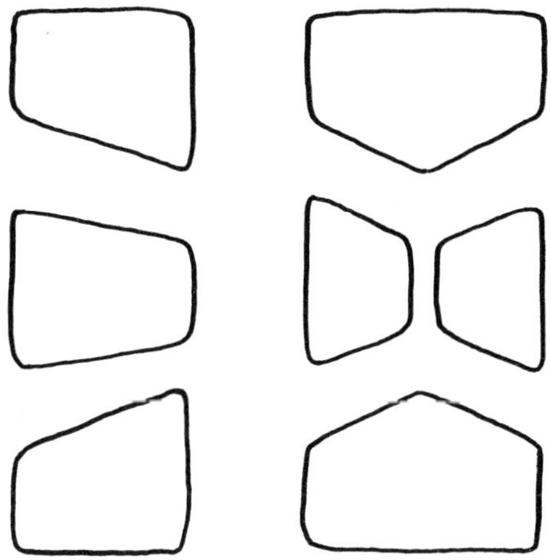

Fig. 5.27

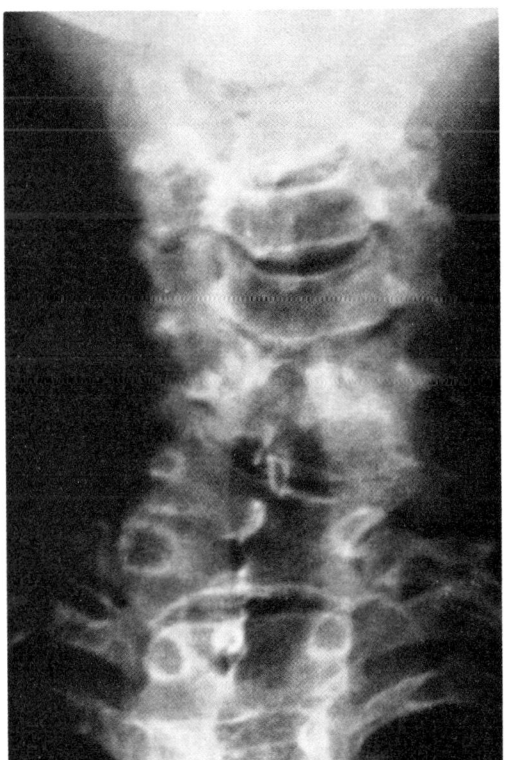

Fig. 5.28 A non-segmented hemi-vertebra on one side is "balanced" by a similar abnormality on the other side. Note gross neurocentral and zygapophyseal osteoarthritis

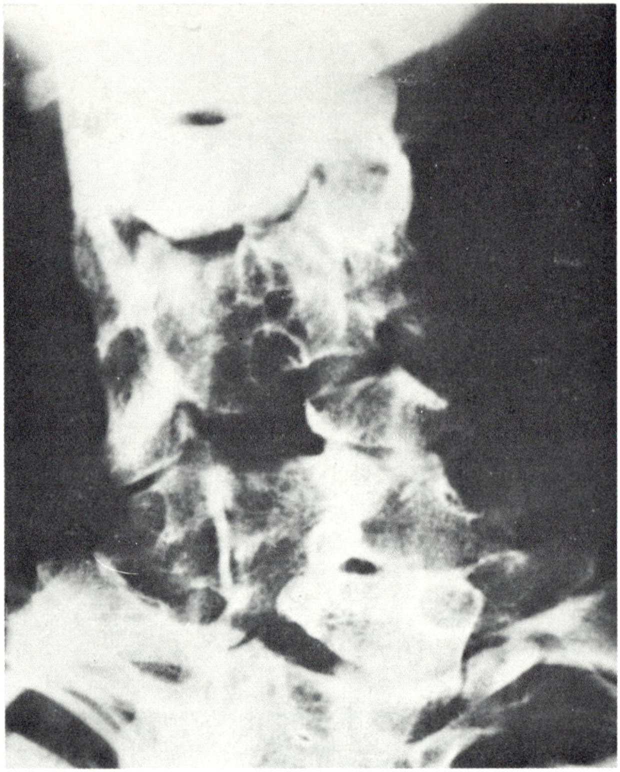

Fig. 5.29 Two hemi-vertebrae on the same side

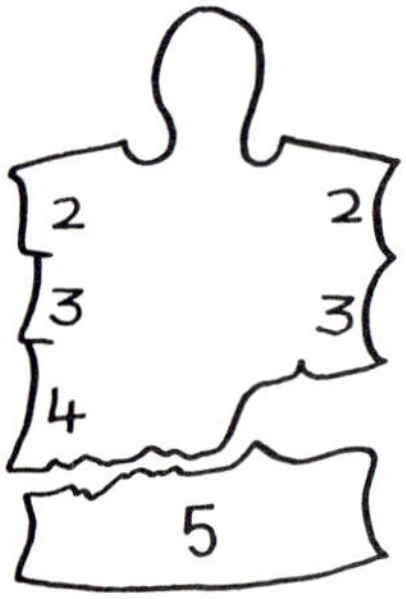

Fig. 5.30

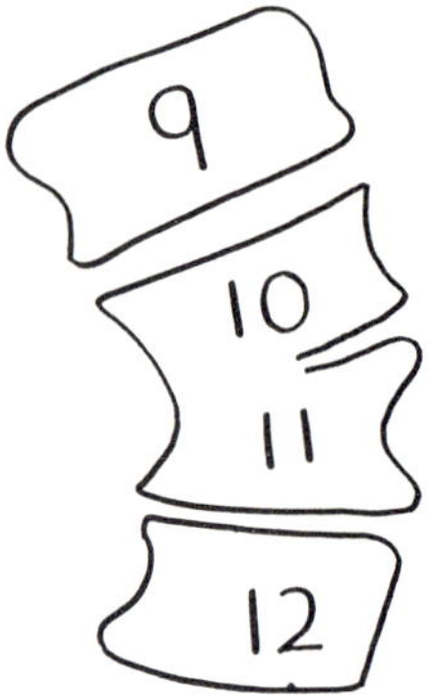

Fig. 5.31

and cord, but if there is lateral dislocation as well, the medulla and cord slide to one side and escape compression.

Non-segmentation Since segmentation precedes ossification, Hadley (1964) prefers to describe congenital union of the vertebrae as non-segmentation rather than fusion. Congenital block vertebrae result from failure of disc formation and may be accompanied by one or more hemi-vertebrae. This abnormality may be unilateral or extend over more segments on one side than the other (Fig. 5.30). The laterally asymmetrical form causes scoliosis (Fig. 5.31). Similarly, anterior fusion causes kyphosis.

The foramina between non-segmented vertebrae have no adjacent joints and have consequently a half moon or oval outline. They are also smaller than normal but are not on this account likely to compress structures contained within them, since they are incapable of being altered in size by movement. Since non-segmentation may be limited to only part of a vertebra the presence of a zygapophyseal joint does not necessarily rebut the diagnosis of non-segmentation, nor on the other hand can union of body and zygapophyseal joint be regarded as being inevitably due to non-segmentation; this can occur in acquired disease as for example in juvenile arthritis, after trauma, disc degeneration, tuberculosis and other infections and in ankylosing spondylosis. Still's disease presents a characteristic appearance in adult life since the vertebrae are of normal height but fail to grow circumferentially. Block vertebrae are frequently associated with gross spondylosis above and below (Fig. 5.25).

In 1964, Gray, Romaine and Skandalis published a collective review and said that congenital fusion of the cervical vertebrae is the common denominator of a galaxy of skeletal defects with poorly known inter-relationships and that one of its best known constellations is the Klippel-Feil Syndrome. The oldest example of congenital cervical vertebral fusion is in an Egyptian mummy of 500 B.C. The abnormality has been recognised since 1559. Other cases were mentioned in the eighteenth and nineteenth centuries, including one by Jonathan Hutchinson Junior (1894). Klippel and Feil (1912) published a complete study of a case of a 46-year-old tailor who died of pneumonia. In 1919 Feil reviewed the entire literature.

The true frequency of the condition is not known. Estimates vary between one in 42,400 births (Luftman and Weintraub, 1951) and three in 700 spinal X-rays (Shands and Bundens, 1956). The anomaly has also been described in the gorilla, so has cervical spondylosis. Gray *et al.* reviewed the fusion in 418 published cases. The sexes are equally affected: females present more commonly during the first year of life, but by the age of 20, 44 per cent of males and 26·5 per cent of females had sought medical attention. Three-quarters of the defects begin in the upper three vertebrae. The extent of the defect tends to be limited at two points. Most of the upper cervical fusions end at the 2nd or 3rd disc level, and most lower cervical defects end at the 6th or 7th disc level. The segment of the 4th and 5th thoracic vertebrae is a similar end point for fusions which extend into the dorsal spine. The other segments of the spine are usually spared.

A single joint was fused in about one-fifth of the cases. The most extreme example showed fusion throughout the spine with only two joints spared—the occipito-cervical and that between the 7th cervical and 1st thoracic vertebra. The non-segmented elements often have a single large spinous process and a single neural arch. One or more cervical ribs are commonly present: there may be atlanto-occipital fusion. Fusion of the sides of the arch may be accompanied by gross spina bifida. It is possible that once the original plan has failed, bony development is modified by the central nervous system. An occipital vertebra occurs when the hypoglossal sclerotome is not assimilated into the skull. Occipitalisation of the atlas occurs when the hypoglossal sclerotome fails to segment from the atlas.

McRae (1960) found that out of 43 cases of occipitalisation of the atlas, 17 showed neurological symptoms, signs or both. It was usually an isolated bony lesion. The anterior end of the assimilated atlas is not only high but also posterior in position. Consequently the odontoid often lies within the foramen magnum. McRae measured the shortest distance from the odontoid to the nearest bony point on the posterior arch of the atlas or the posterior lip of the foramen magnum. Symptoms or signs were found in all cases in which this was less than 19 mm. An occipital vertebra may be partly fused to the foramen magnum. Atlanto-occipital fusion may be unilateral and may be associated with basilar impression. Non-segmentation below the fused atlas may produce torticollis. Congenital anomalies at the atlanto-occipital junction are not always fully demonstrated in plain lateral films. In all upper cord lesions, in torticollis and in patients with asymmetry of the head and neck, a full forward flexion lateral film must be taken.

Basilar invagination enters into the differential diagnosis of lesions at the cranio-vertebral junction and may be mistaken for occipitalisation of the atlas. Antero-posterior and lateral tomography are necessary to show that neither the lateral mass nor the arch of the atlas are fused to the skull. The lines of Chamberlain (1939) and McGregor (1948) may be misleading owing to the variability of the plane of the foramen magnum and the prominence and slope of the occipital condyles. In basilar invagination the occipital condyles move upwards into the base of the skull taking the atlas with them. Since the articular surfaces of the atlas are placed anteriorly the displacement of the occipital condyles imparts an upward tilt to the anterior extremity of the atlas. Bull *et al.* (1955) has related this tilt to the comparatively stable line of the hard palate. Two lines are drawn, one along the hard palate and another from the middle of the anterior arch of the atlas to the middle of its posterior arch as seen in a lateral radiograph. When this angle exceeds 10 degrees primary basilar impression should be suspected.

Congenital torticollis Gyorgyi (1965) examined 20 cases of congenital torticollis and observed a variety of co-existing abnormalities including spondylosis, asymmetry of the zygapophyseal condyles, basilar impression, atlanto-axial dislocation, occipitalisation of the atlas, synostosis between the lateral mass of the atlas and the body of the axis, and aplasia or deformity of the odontoid process. Congenital torticollis also leads to early spondylosis (as shown in Fig. 5.32). In 40 per cent of these patients there was a history of breech presentation. There is also an association between breech presentation and congenital dislocation of the hip. Andren (1962), discussing this, suggested that the factors producing congenital dislocation of the hip in the child influence the maternal uterus in such a way as to predispose to breech presentation. Perhaps a similar mechanism affects the cervical spine.

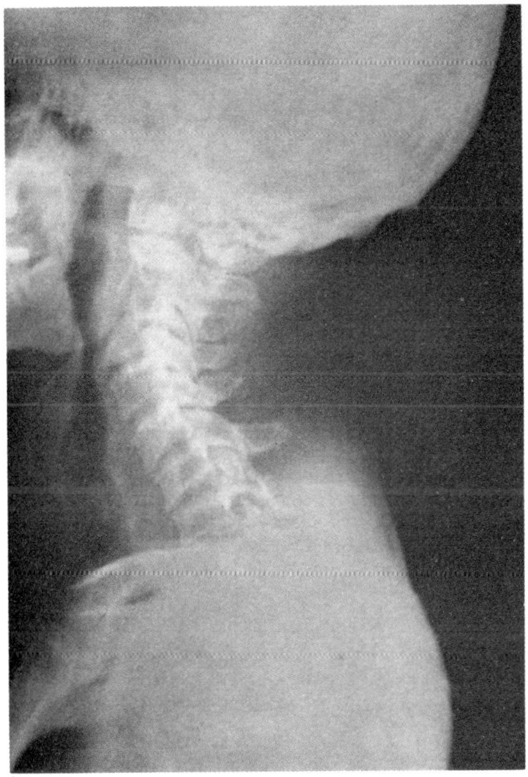

Fig. 5.32 Congenital spasmodic torticollis leading to severe cervical spondylosis at the age of 37

Rheumatoid arthritis

Sharp *et al.* (1958) defined the radiological changes produced in the cervical spine by rheumatoid arthritis (R.A.) in adults and show that these changes may be the only evidence of R.A.

They found narrowing of disc spaces, often multiple, affecting the discs C2–3 and C3–4 more often than others. Disc narrowing was not particularly associated with osteophytes. The vertebral plates, instead of being sclerosed, tended to be eroded. Vertebral subluxation of more than a "mild degree" affected the bodies adjacent to the diseased discs; the atlanto-axial joint may also be involved. (Atlanto-axial movement of 8 mm was recorded in one patient.) Erosion of zygapophyseal joints also occurs but in the series reported by these authors this was difficult to assess, since only a lateral view of the cervical spine was available. One of the important points to emerge from this study is the possibility of radiological change in rheumatoid arthritis being restricted to the cervical spine.

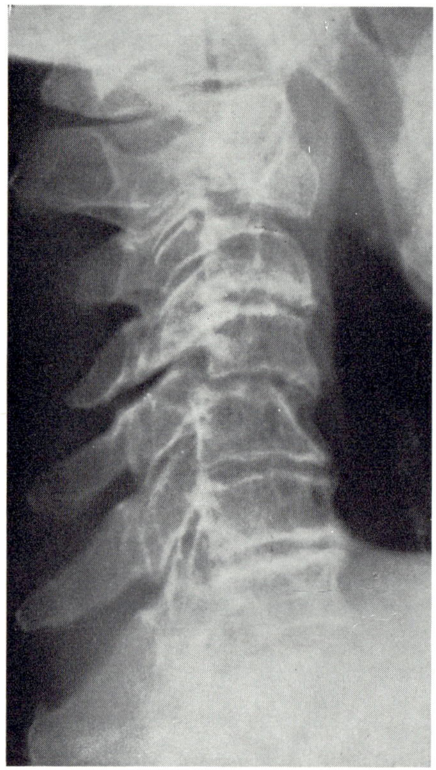

Fig. 5.33 Gross narrowing, erosion and forward subluxation in rheumatoid arthritis. Note spondylosis at C6–7

Bland *et al.* (1963) added the following points: platysbasia may occur: there is generalised osteoporosis: osteosclerosis may be seen in the atlanto-axial-occipital area. Eighty-six per cent of the patients with classified R.A.* had evidence of cervical spine involvement. This seems to be an extremely high figure but the authors were using a very careful radiographic technique.

In reading the literature it should be borne in mind that the Americans have been

* American Rheumatism Association.

reluctant to accept the separation of rheumatoid spondylitis into spondylitis due to rheumatoid arthritis and that due to ankylosing spondylitis, a distinction which has been accepted in this country for some time.

Conlon *et al.* (1966) drew attention to the value of tomography in the diagnosis of atlanto-axial subluxation. They examined 333 patients with R.A., using a lateral film in full flexion. They found that 50 necks were normal, 106 showed zygapophyseal erosion or blurring, 84 showed atlanto-axial subluxation and 23 showed serious subluxation.

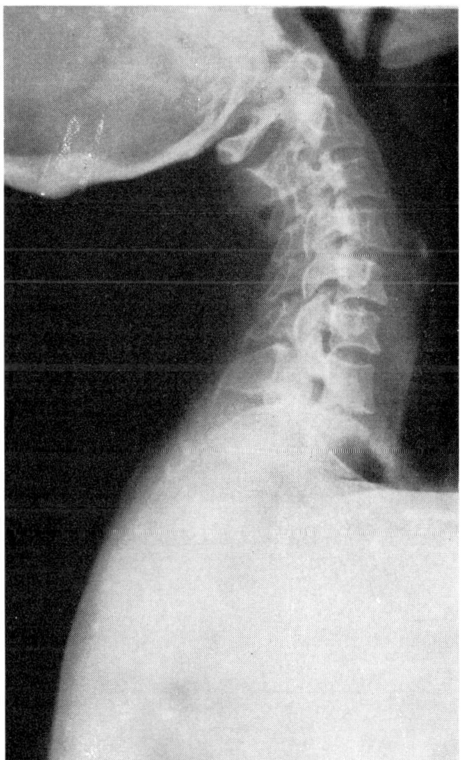

Fig. 5.34 Even in extension there is forward subluxation of several bodies (rheumatoid arthritis)

Disc narrowing without osteophytosis occurred in 59 patients and vertebral end-plate erosion in 48. One patient showed platybasia and there were 8 examples each of spinous process erosion and odontoid erosion.

Figure 5.33 shows the characteristic forward subluxation and gross narrowing of the upper discs, especially at C3–4. The appearances at C5–6 with sclerosis and osteophytosis suggest concomitant spondylosis. Forward subluxation may be present even in films taken in extension in rheumatoid arthritis. Figure 5.34 shows this atlanto-axial subluxation. The appearances are dramatic in flexion. The almost isolated gross atlanto-axial dislocation is illustrated in Figure 5.35. Figure 5.36 shows erosion of the odontoid in rheumatoid arthritis and subluxation at C3–4. In Lawrence's classification, mentioned above, intermediate rheumatoid arthritis appears to be associated with painful arthrosis of the zygapophyseal joints. It is clear from his paper that various kinds of evidence including serology are necessary to differentiate arthrosis which is secondary to rheumatoid arthritis from arthrosis which is apparent primary.

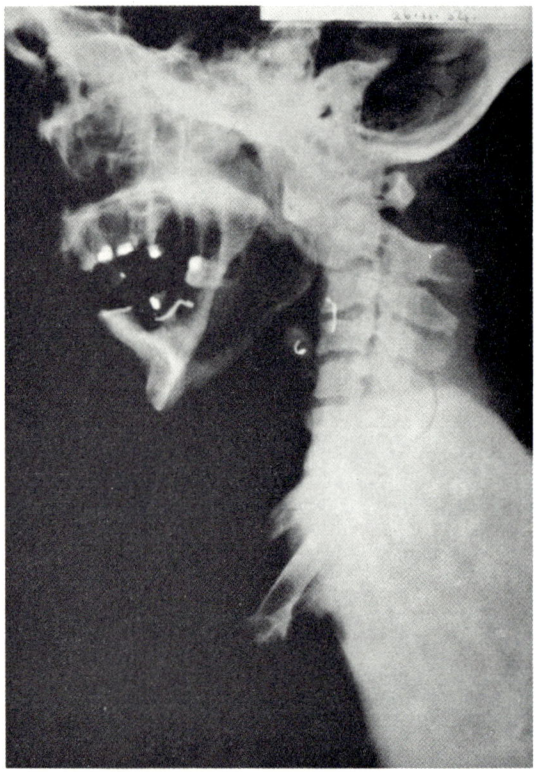

Fig. 5.35 Gross atlanto-axial displacement in rheumatoid arthritis

Still's Disease—Juvenile Rheumatoid Arthritis

In his original communication Still (1897) mentioned the early involvement of the cervical spine in patients with juvenile rheumatoid arthritis. Middlemiss (1951) observed that the zygapophyseal joints are first affected and this leads to ankylosis.

Ziff *et al.* (1958) describe their findings in 16 patients, 12 of whom show isolated spinal changes. Of these the most characteristic appearance is fusion of the zygapophyseal joints at C2–3 and less often at C3–4 or even lower. They describe loss of lordosis, even kyphosis, underdevelopment of bodies and thinning of discs. (They do not mention fusion of bodies but this is apparent in their illustration.)

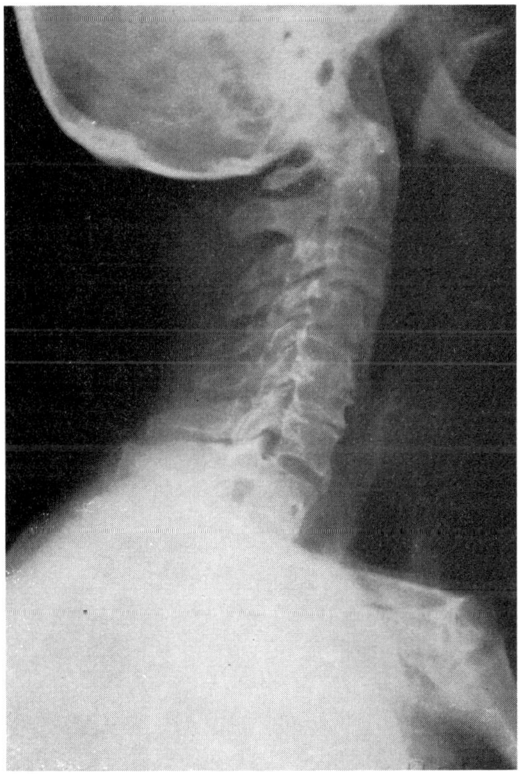

Fig. 5.36 In rheumatoid arthritis the odontoid may be eroded and there is a narrowing and subluxation, especially of the upper cervical discs (note C3–4). The discs C5–6 and C6–7 show additional degenerative changes but there is erosion of the vertebral end plates and the disc narrowing is extensive in relation to the sclerosis

Underdevelopment of the bodies of the vertebrae occurs in chronic arthritis after recurrent rheumatic fever and ankylosing spondylitis of early onset. The bodies are restricted in their antero-posterior diameter but apparently grow to a normal height.

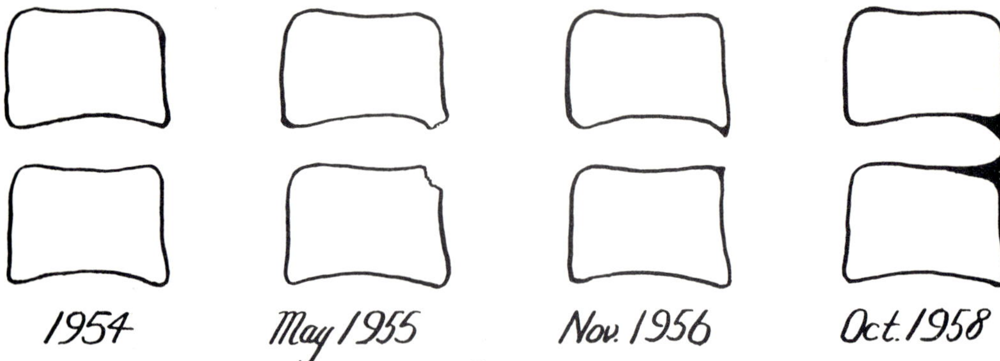

Fig. 5.37

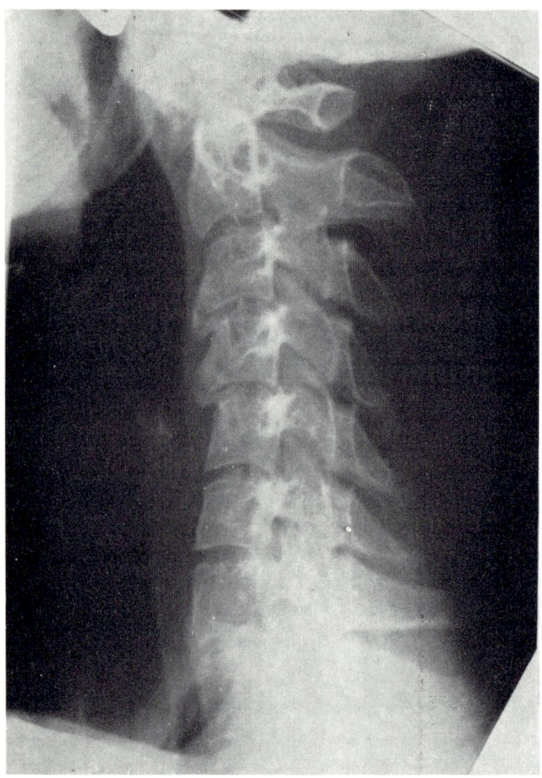

Fig. 5.38a Subluxation occurring in ankylosing spondylitis

Rheumatic Fever

Thomas (1956) in describing the joint changes following recurrent rheumatoid fever mentions the irregularity and fusion of the zygapophyseal joints, narrowing of the discs and increased height of the vertebral bodies. His illustration suggests that it is not the height that is abnormal but the antero-posterior diameter. He also describes ossification in the discs. All his patients had valvular disease of the heart.

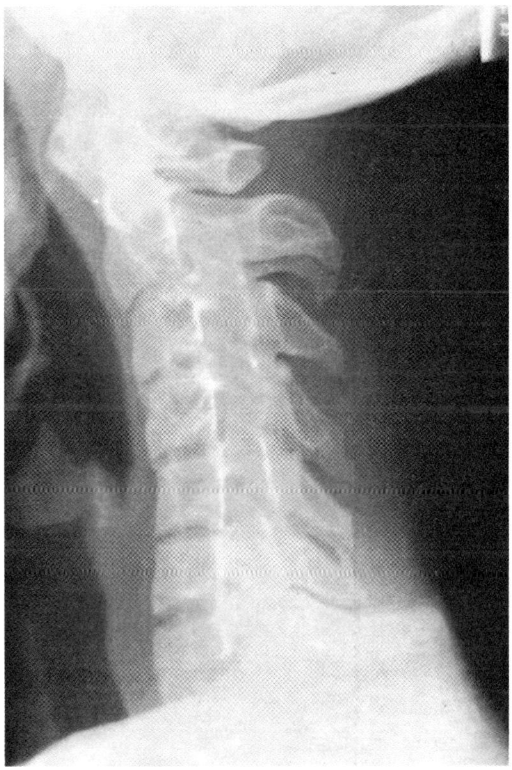

Fig. 5.38b A film taken a few years later shows fusion of the zygapophyseal joints with reduction of the subluxation

Ankylosing Spondylitis

When the cervical spine is affected in patients with ankylosing spondylitis, it shows the characteristic march of events seen in the sacro-iliac joints: erosion, sclerosis and ankylosis. The chronological sequence is illustrated in Figure 5.37. The process involves the anterior angles of the vertebral bodies shown in the lateral view; the bony

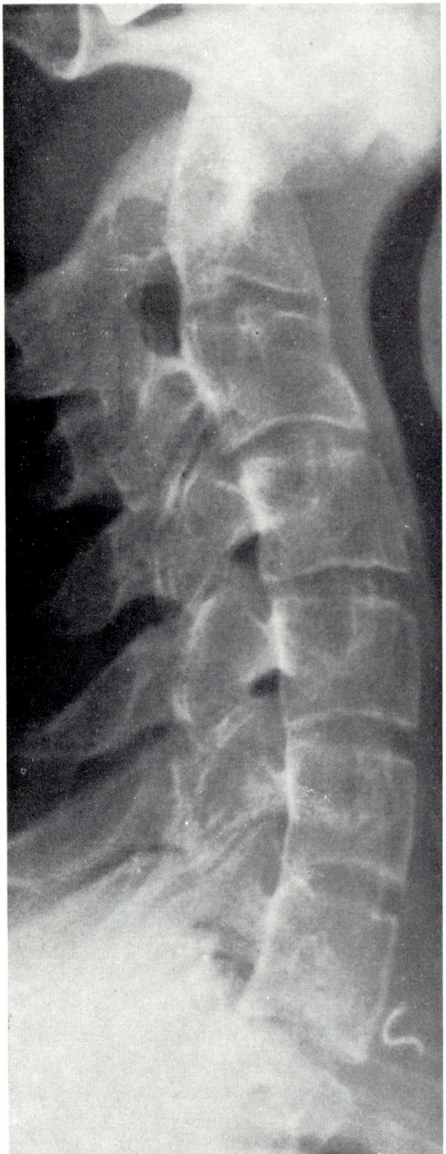

Fig. 5.39 Gross subluxation of the atlanto-axial joint in ankylosing spondylitis. The characteristic changes are seen in the lower cervical vertebrae with ankylosis between the bodies of C2–3, erosion of the anterior upper angle of the body of C5 and squaring of the upper anterior angle of the body of C6

spurs which form are directed upwards or downwards and not horizontally as in cervical spondylosis. Similar changes also occur in the neurocentral and in the zygapophyseal joints. The discs are preserved but there may be very marked subluxation which later becomes fixed by the process of ossification (Fig. 5.38a and b). During this process of "fixing" the subluxation may become reduced. The joint between the odontoid and the arch of the atlas may be severely involved with a major degree of subluxation (Fig. 5.39) but the erosion and sclerosis here (well seen tomographically in Fig. 5.11) and characteristic changes elsewhere lead to a correct diagnosis.

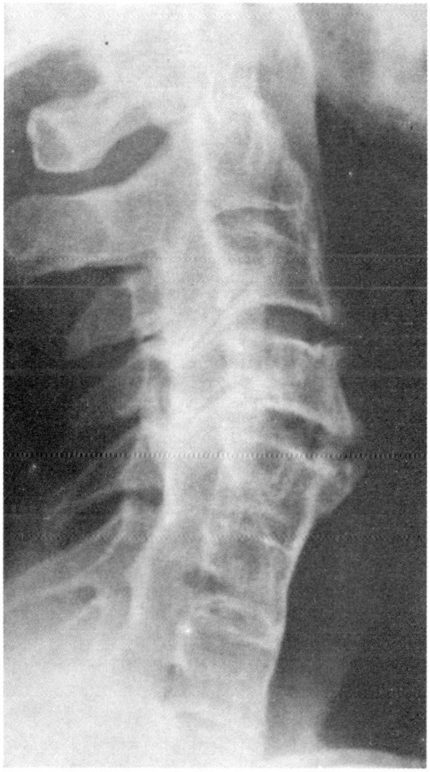

Fig. 5.40 Gross zygapophyseal degeneration in the joints adjacent to vertebrae fused by ankylosing spondylitis

Even if some of the vertebral joints are spared they may degenerate early (Fig. 5.40). To this extent it is possible that ankylosing spondylosis can predispose to local spondylosis. In the example illustrated, osteophyte formation is very marked and zygapophyseal osteophytes could be seen even in the A.P. view.

During the investigation of patients with ankylosing spondylitis or rheumatoid arthritis, radiography of the sacro-iliac joints and of the extremities should not be neglected, Mason *et al.* (1959). Sacro-iliitis also occurs in psoriatic arthropathy, ulcerative colitis, Crohn's disease and Reiter's disease and concomitant changes in the cervical spine can only be interpreted against the background of the clinical picture.

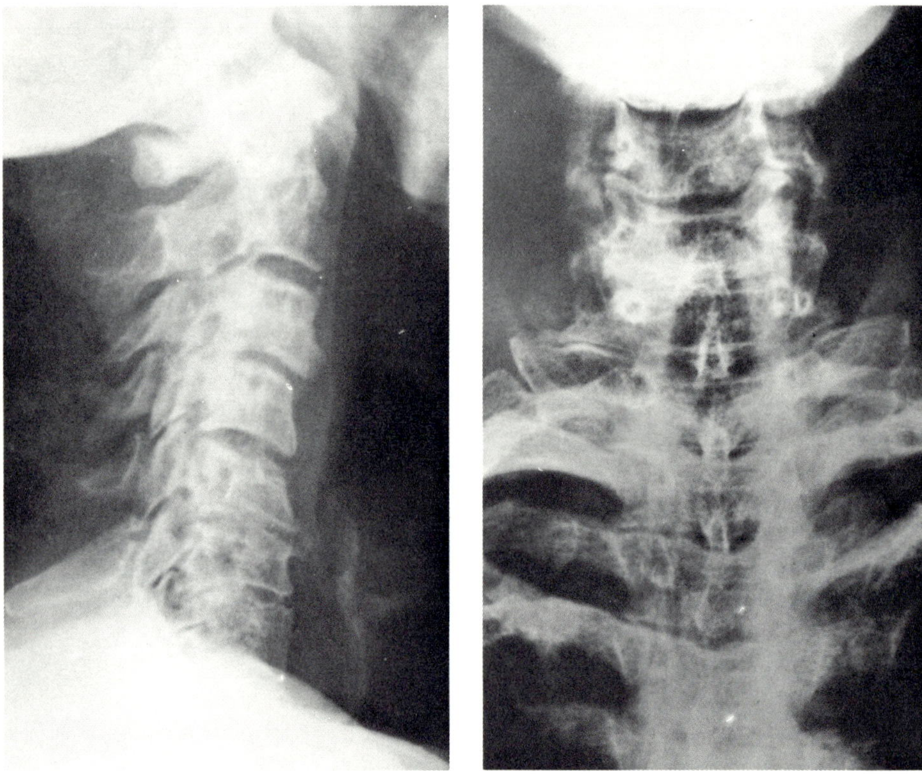

Fig. 5.41a and b Lateral and A.P. films of patient suffering from tabes dorsalis. The discs are narrowed; there is gross osteophytosis with forward subluxation of the bodies. The lower bodies are also compressed

Cervical Arthropathy

This term includes the changes in the cervical spine occurring in tabes dorsalis, diabetes and syringomyelia. Radiographic examination shows very severe florid and rapidly progressive changes which are similar to those of cervical spondylosis of a very marked kind. There is a tendency for more bone destruction in arthropathy and for osteophytes to be larger and more irregular than usual (Fig. 5.41a and b and Fig. 5.42a and b).

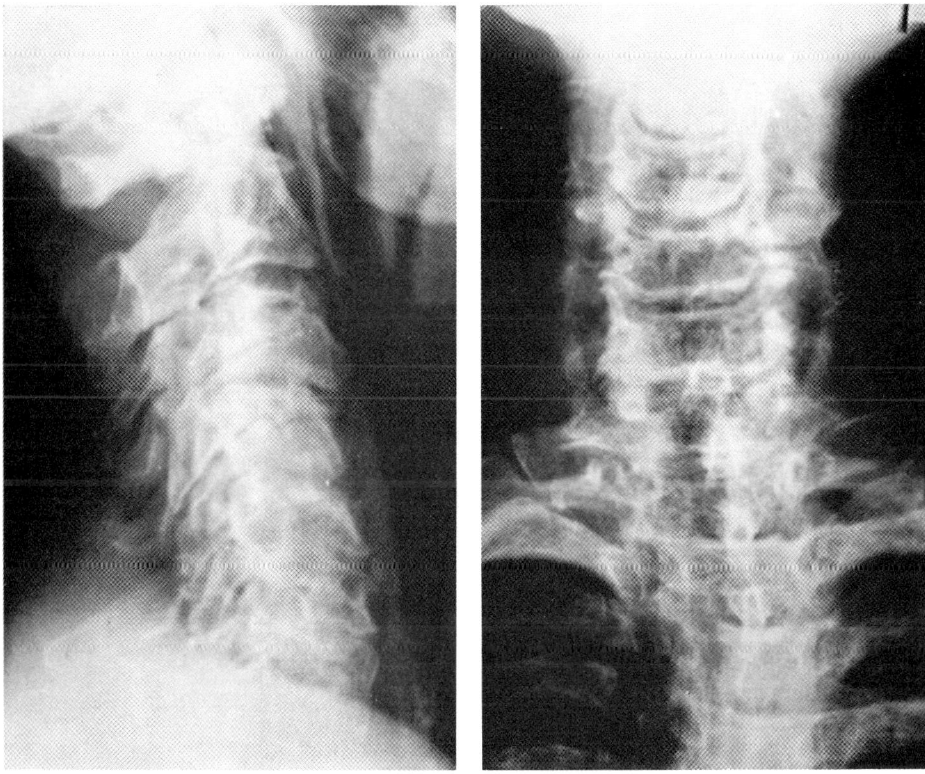

Fig. 5.42a and b Films of the same patient 4 years later. The changes have progressed rapidly. The zygapophyseal joints are grossly abnormal. All the discs, except C2–3, are narrow and there is gross sclerosis. The appearances are typical of cervical arthropathy

Gout

This will very rarely present a problem in radiological differential diagnosis. Patients with gout may suffer from spinal pain due to urate deposits but X-ray films are usually negative. Subluxation of the atlas has occurred and there may be tophaceous invasion of vertebral bodies. Myelography may show filling defects in the spinal canal.

Steroid Arthropathy

Steroid treatment may lead to changes in the cervical spine as in other joints. In the example shown (Fig. 5.43) there is gross subluxation of the bodies and destruction of the upper zygapophyseal joints.

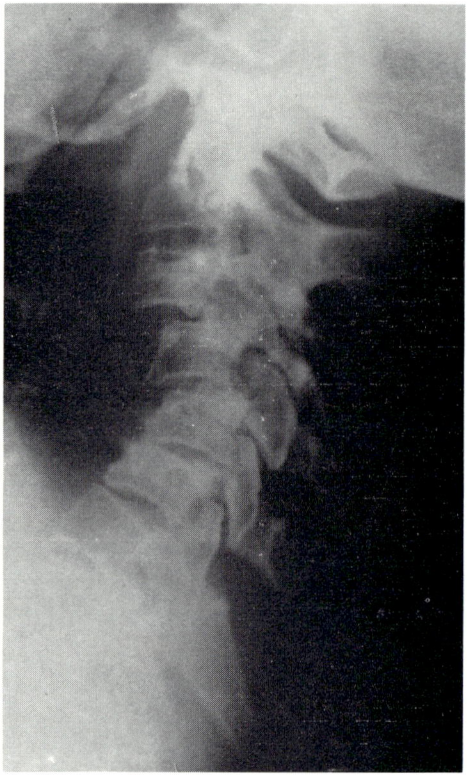

Fig. 5.43 Steroid arthropathy—the degenerative changes are relatively mild but there is gross subluxation in flexion, especially between C3–4. The appearances are reminiscent of the changes of rheumatoid arthritis

Traumatic Lesions

The spinous process of the 7th cervical vertebra can be fractured directly or more often by muscular violence. A sudden twisting or jerking movement of the neck may strain the inter-articular ligaments without actually displacing or dislocating the joints. Symptoms are caused by oedema and haemorrhage round the adjacent nerve roots. It is essential that a lateral view is taken with the spine fully flexed in order to exclude sub-luxation or dislocation. Sub-luxation of the interarticular joints is differentiated from dislocation in that the articular processes have not overridden. This may occur as a minor factor in a traumatic situation, but if it is not recognised by the use of extension and flexion films, neurological sequelae may persist. It may occur during the

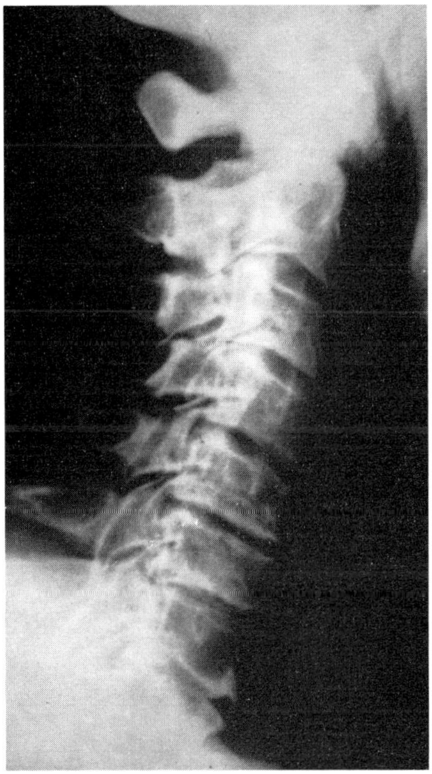

Fig. 5.44 Paget's Disease. The lower cervical bodies are elongated and compressed. The trabecular pattern is coarse and there is a patchy increase of density. Degenerative lipping is also present and the lower discs are narrowed due to concomittant spondylosis

involuntary forward jerk when a car stops suddenly. The true cause of symptoms in such cases may not be known for several years after the event which, by that time, may have been forgotten. Patients with the grosser forms of cervical trauma are unlikely to attend the physician in the first instance and the changes are, in any case, only too obvious in the lateral view.

Fractures and dislocations of the atlas usually occur as a result of severe trauma so that the history is unequivocal, but dislocation of the atlas does occur with nearby infection in the neck, also in rheumatoid arthritis and sometimes in ankylosing spondylitis.

INFLAMMATORY DISORDERS

Pyogenic infection As has already been stated, local sepsis in the neck can give rise to

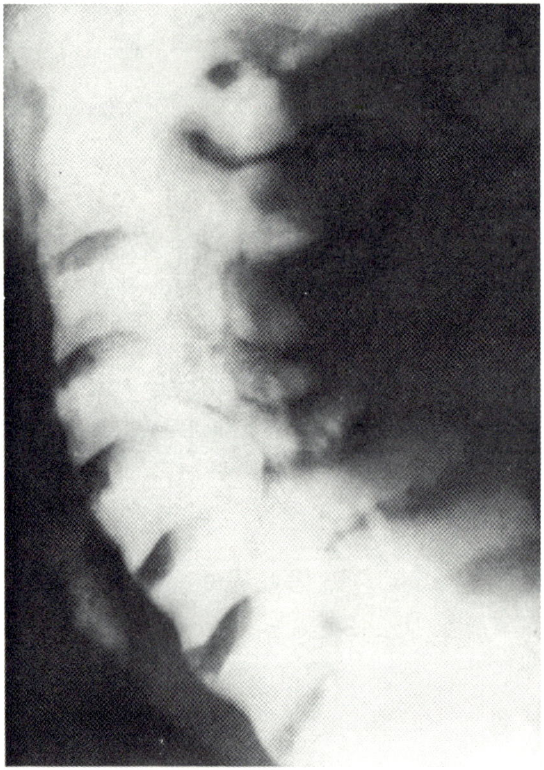

Fig. 5.45 Fluorosis. The vertebrae are uniformly dense. There are bony projections on the anterior aspects of the bodies passing upwards and downwards rather than horizontally and fusing in at least two places. These spurs do not resemble those of spondylosis. There are also bony projections from the spinous process

dislocation of the vertebrae but this is probably not due to extension of the infection but rather to softening of ligaments consequent upon increased vascularity. Pyogenic osteomyelitis of the cervical spine is uncommon. Tuberculosis, however, still occurs although less frequently in the cervical than in other parts of the spine. In the early stages of pyogenic and tuberculous osteomyelitis bone destruction occurs in the region

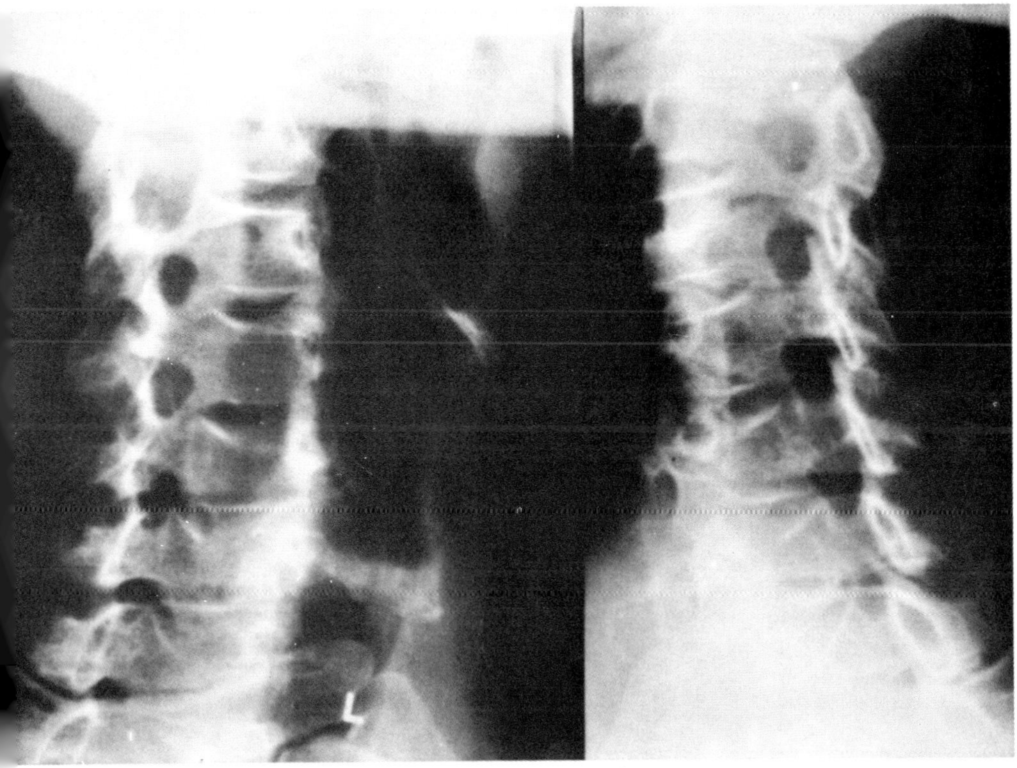

Fig. 5.46 Gross enlargement of the foramen C2–3 by neurofibroma

of the vertebral plate and spreads across the disc to involve the adjacent vertebra. It is followed by narrowing of the cervical disc. This progresses more rapidly in pyogenic osteomyelitis as does bone proliferation and the appearance of sclerosis, but in tuberculous lesions it takes 6 months for sclerotic changes to develop, if indeed they ever do. Thus, from the radiological point of view, the differential diagnosis between the two depends upon serial films. Salmonella osteomyelitis can present a real difficulty since there is a relation between salmonella infection and sickle cell anemia. Radiological changes may be delayed for 4–8 weeks after the onset of symptoms and only repeated examination may demonstrate changes. Some 4 to 6 weeks after the first radiological signs new bone appears in the body or bodies, and is seen as spur formation. The end result is fusion of adjacent bodies. The disease may be limited to the

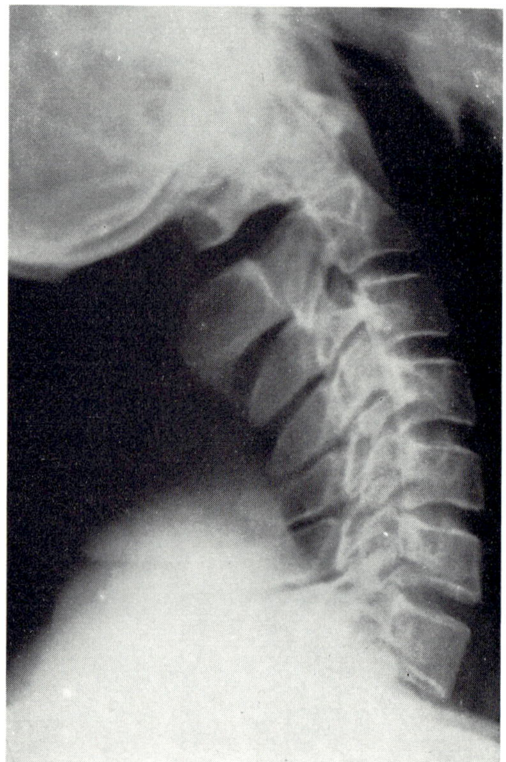

Fig. 5.47 As in Fig. 5.46; note appearance in lateral view

odontoid process. Brucellosis may cause extensive destruction of bodies and discs especially in young people, but in general the changes are proliferative with little alteration of contour of bone.

Tuberculosis The cervical spine is less commonly affected than the dorsal and lumbar regions. The earliest sign is usually decalcification of the upper or lower aspect of a vertebral body, but central or anterior defects may be the presenting lesion. The body then collapses, the discs become disrupted and infected. The end result is wedging of one or more bodies with fusion. Abscesses may involve adjacent tissues and later shows the characteristic calcification.

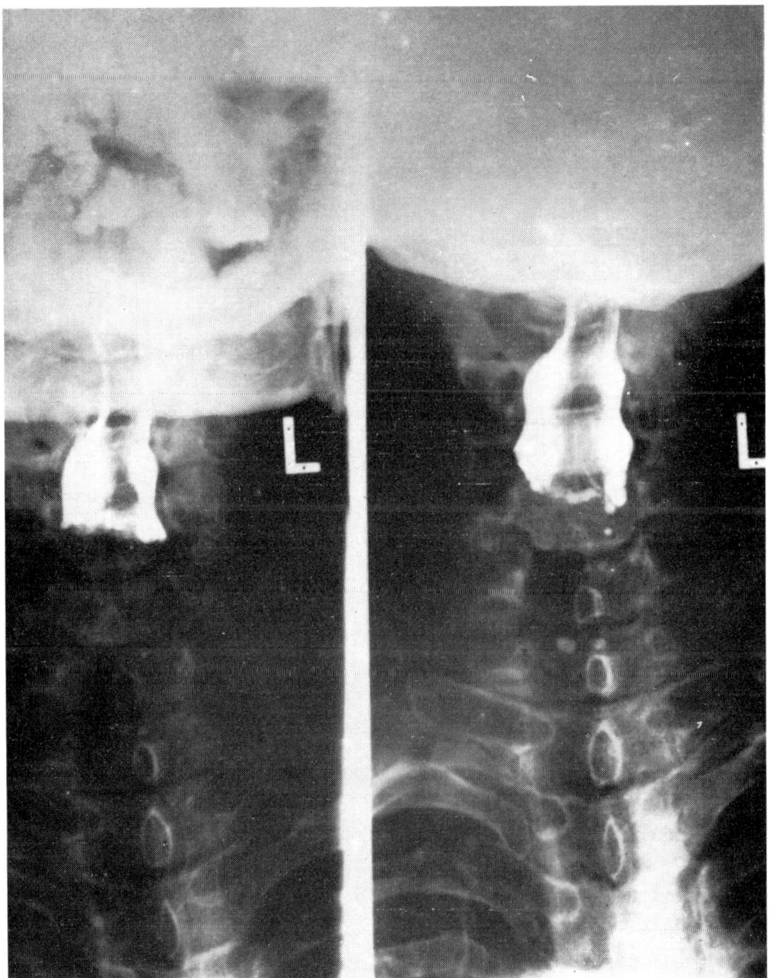

Fig. 5.48 Typical appearance in a myelogram of extradural tumour. Neurofibroma at C2–3

Syphilis The lesion is gummatous, and may affect one or more vertebrae. It is intensely painful and very destructive. The anterior aspects of bodies are most severely involved, but the whole of the vertebra, including the spinous process may show a "moth eaten" appearance. Proliferative changes are sparse. After treatment the bone regenerates and the vertebrae become fused with bizarre deformities.

Paget's disease The cervical spine is relatively rarely involved in this condition which may affect one or more vertebrae. It occasionally leads to compression of the spinal cord. The earliest radiological sign is increased density of the vertebrae sometimes with increased vertical trabecular markings. The increased density may be

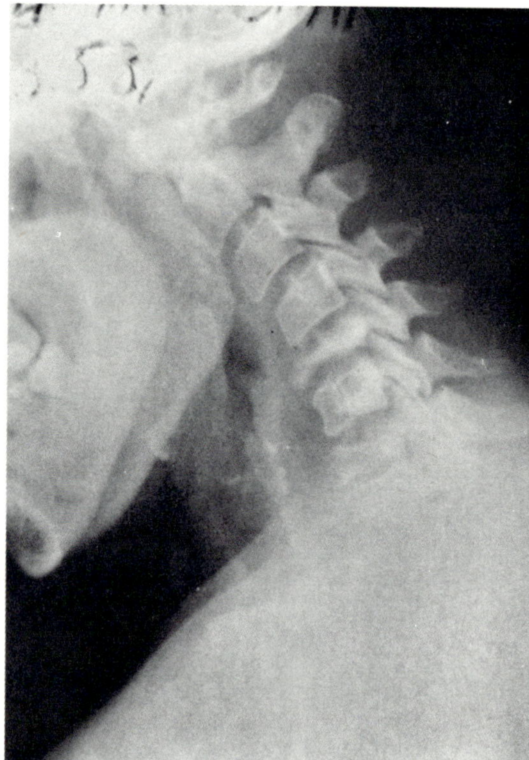

Fig. 5.49 Destruction of the body of C5 by metastasis. C7 is also involved

patchy, rather like osteoblastic metastasis (Fig. 5.44). In some cases the body becomes uniformly opaque; the so called "ivory vertebra". When this is seen the possibilities of metastasis (especially from the prostate) and Hodgkin's disease should be borne in mind. Staphylococcal infection can, rarely, produce this appearance.

As Paget's disease progresses the vertebra becomes a little flattened and there may be involvement of the adnexae. The trabecular pattern becomes coarse and the affected parts of the bone widened. In patients with spondylosis the earliest changes of Paget's disease begin in the osteophytes.

Fluorosis In this condition there is patchy or diffuse sclerosis of all or part of the vertebrae. The diffuse changes are accompanied by bony outgrowth (Fig. 5.45).

NEOPLASMS OF BONE

Theoretically any bony neoplasm can occur in the cervical spine but from the practical point of view these are rare and are unlikely to cause confusion in the diagnosis of cervical spondylosis. Among the possibilities angioma and giant cell tumour are occasionally encountered.

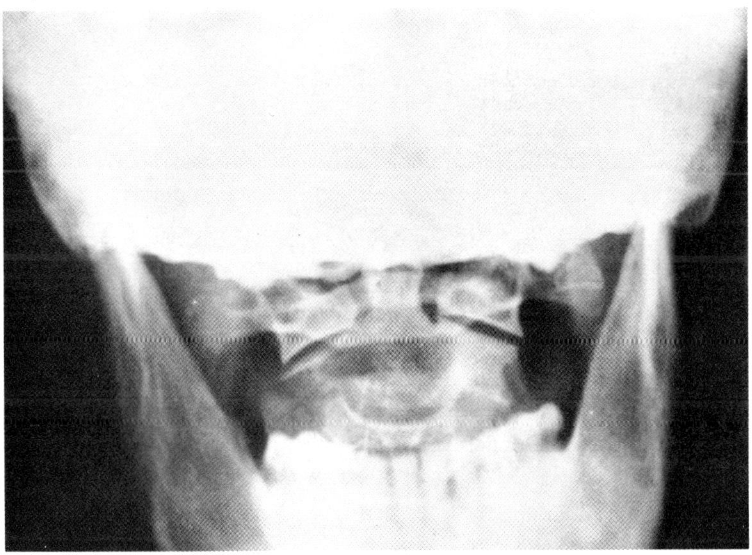

Fig. 5.50 A.P. view of same patient, note destruction of lateral mass

Neurofibroma This is a less rare tumour which may very occasionally cause confusion. It is worth bearing in mind since it might be responsible for some of the symptoms and signs in a patient with cervical spondylosis. It characteristically causes enlargement of the intervertebral foramen. In the example illustrated (in Figs. 5.46 and 5.47) a large defect can be seen not only in the oblique view but also in the lateral view. The diagnosis is confirmed myelographically (Fig. 5.48).

Secondary carcinomas These are usually destructive and part of the vertebrae may be involved. Classically the body (Fig. 5.49) or several bodies are partly destroyed.

Diagnosis is not difficult especially as the discs tend to be spared. When one body is involved the possibility of infection arises. If only part of the vertebra, for example the lateral mass (Fig. 5.50) is destroyed careful radiography and perhaps tomography is necessary.

Sclerotic secondary deposits (Fig. 5.51) may be mistaken for Paget's disease, Hodgkin's disease, fluorosis, staphylococcal infection and myeloma.

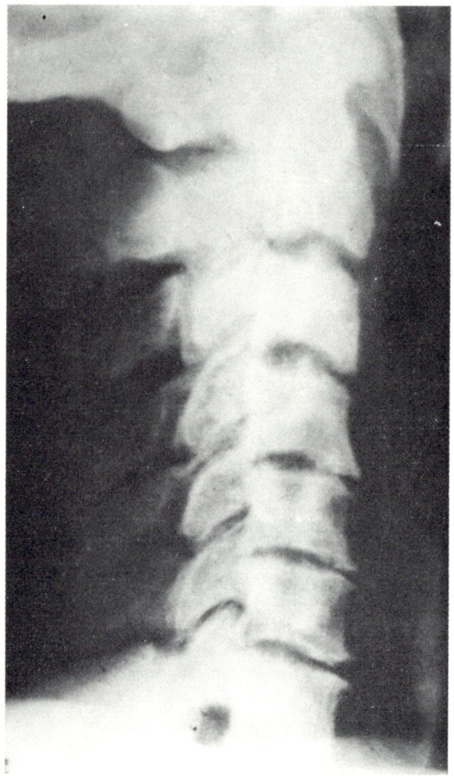

Fig. 5.51 Secondary deposits from carcinoma of the prostate. There are some changes of spondylosis but there is also patchy sclerosis of the bodies

References

Andrén, L. (1962), "Pelvic instability in newborns", *Acta radiol., Stockh.*, Suppl. 212.

Bailey, D. K. (1952), "The normal cervical spine in infants and children", Radiology, **59**, 712.

Bland, J. H., Davis, P. H., London, M. G., Van Buskirk, F. W. and Duarte, C. G. (1963), "Rheumatoid arthritis of cervical spine", *Arch. intern. Med.*, **112**, 892.

Brain, W. R. (1963), "Some unsolved problems of cervical spondylosis, *Brit. med. J.*, **1**, 771.

Bull, J. W. D. (1948), "Discussion on rupture of the intervertebral disc in the cervical region", *Proc. R. Soc. Med.*, **41**, 513.

Bull, J. W. D., Nixon, W. L. B. and Pratt, R. T. C. (1955), "The radiological criteria and familial occurrence of primary basilar impression", *Brain*, **78**, 229.

Chamberlain, W. E. (1939), "Basilar impression (platybasia): a bizarre developmental anomaly of the occipital bone and upper cervical spine with striking and misleading neurologic manifestations", *Yale J. Biol. Med.*, **11**, 487.

Coliez, R. T. (1965), "Anatomie radiologique des trous de conjugaison cervicaux (Rappel)", *J. Radiol. Electrol.*, **46**, 437.

Conlon, P. W., Isdale, I. C. and Rose, B. S. (1966), "Rheumatoid arthritis of the cervical spine", *Ann. rheum. Dis.*, **25**, 120.

Council for International Organizations of Medical Sciences (1963), "The epidemiology of chronic rheumatism", Vol. I edited by J. H. Kellgren, M. R. Jeffrey and J. Ball, Oxford.

Crandall, P. H. and Hanafee, W. N. (1964), "Cervical spondylotic myelopathy studied by air myelography", *Amer. J. Roentenol.*, **92**, 1260.

Dugan, M. C., Locke, S. and Gallagher, J. R. (1962), "Occipital neuralgia in adolescents and young adults", *New Engl. J. Med.*, **267**, 1166.

Feil, A. (1919), "L'absence et la diminution des vertèbres cervicales (étude clinique et pathogénique), Thesis, Paris.

Feinberg, S. B. (1964), "The place of diskography in radiology as based on 2,320 cases", *Amer. J. Roentgenol.*, **92**, 1275.

Gould, P. L., Peyton, W. T. and French, L. A. (1955), "Vertebral angiography by retrograde injection of the brachial artery", *J. Neurosurg.*, **12**, 369.

Grainger, R. G. (1960), In "Modern trends in diagnostic radiology" (Third series), Ed. by J. W. McLaren, London, p. 260.

Gray, S. W., Romaine, C. B. and Skandalakis, J. E. (1964), "Congenital fusion of the cervical vertebrae", *Surg. Gynec., Obstet.*, **118**, 373.

Gyorgyi, G. (1965), "Les changements morphologiques de la region occipito-cervicale associés au torticolis", *J. Radiol. Electrol.*, **45**, 797

Hadley, L. A. (1956), "The spine; anatomico-radiographic studies", Thomas, Springfield.

Holt, E. P. Jr. (1964), "Fallacy of cervical discography", *J. Amer. med., Ass.*, **188**, 799.

Hutchinson, J. Jr. (1894), "Deformity of shoulder girdle", *Brit. med. J.*, **1**, 634.

James, J. L. (1965), "The treatment of myelopathy due to cervical spondylosis", Thesis, Bristol University.

Juhl, J. H., Miller, S. M. and Roberts, G. W. (1962), "Roentgenographic variations in the normal cervical spine", *Radiology*, **78**, 591.

Klippel, M., and Feil, A. (1912a), "Anomalie de la colonne vertébrale par absence des vertebres cervicales—cage thoracique remontant jusqu'à la base du crâne", *Bull. Soc. anat. Paris*, **87**, 185.

Klippel, M. and Feil, A. (1912b), "Un cas d'absence des vertèbres cervicales avec cage thoracique remontant jusqu'à la base du crâne (cage thoracique cervicale)", *Noust. Iconogr. Salpêt.*, **25**, 223.

Klippel, M. and Feil, A. (1912c), "Absence de colonne cervicale, Cage thoracique remontant jusqu'à la base du crâne", *Pr. méd.*, **20**, 411.

Klippel, M. and Feil, A. (1912d), "Un cas d'absence des vertèbres cervicales, cage thoracique remontant jusqu'à la base due crâne", *Bull. Soc. anthrop. Paris*, **65**, 101.

Kovács, A. (1955). "Subluxation and deformation of the cervical apophyseal joints", *Acta radiol., Stockh.*, **43**, 1.

Kuhn, R. A. (1960), "The normal brachial cerebral angiogram", *Amer. J. Roentgenol.*, **84**, 78.

Lawrence, J. S., de Graaff, R. and Laine, V. A. I. (1963), *In* Council for International Organizations of Medical Sciences, the Epidemiology of Chronic Rheumatism, Vol. I, edited by J. H. Kellgren, M. R. Jeffrey and J. Ball, Oxford, p. 98.

Lawrence, J. S. Bremner, J. M. and Bier, F. (1966), "Osteo-arthrosis: prevalence in the population and relationship between symptoms and X-ray changes", *Ann. rheum. Dis.*, **25**, 1.

Lindgren, E. (1950), "Percutaneous angiography of the vertebral artery", *Acta. radiol., Stockh.*, **33**, 389.

Luftman, I. I. and Weintraub, S. (1951), "Klippel-Feil syndrome in a full-term stillborn infant", *N.Y. Ct. J. Med.*, **51**, 2035.

McGregor, M. (1948), "The significance of certain measurements of the skull in the diagnosis of basilar impression", *Brit. J. Radiol.*, **21**, 171.

McRae, D. L. (1956), "Asymptomatic intervertebral disc protrusions", *Acta radiol., Stockh.*, **46**, 9.

McRae, D. L. (1960), "The significance of abnormalities of the cervical spine", *Amer. J. Roentgenol.*, **84**, 3.

Mason, R. M., Murray, R. S., Oates, J. K. and Young, A. C. (1959), "A comparative radiological study of Reiter's disease, rheumatoid arthritis and ankylosing spondylitis", *J. Bone Jt. Surg.*, **41–3**, 137.

Middlemiss, J. H. (1951), "Juvenile rheumatoid arthritis", (Still's disease), *Proc. R. Soc. Med.*, **44**, 805.

Niemyer, T. and Penning L. (1963), "Functional roentgenographic examination in a case of cervical spondylolisthesis", *J. Bone Jt. Surg.*, **45–A**, 1671.

Pallis, C., Jones, A. M. and Spillane, J. D. (1954), "Cervical spondylosis, incidence and implication", *Brain*, **77**, 274.

Paris, F. A. and Young, A. C. (1967).

Payne, E. E. (1959), "The cervical spine and spondylosis", *Neurochirurgia*, **1**, 178.

Penning, L. (1964), "Nonpathologic and pathologic relationships between the lower cervical vertebrae", *Amer. J. Roentgenol.*, **91**, 1036.

Pygott, F. and Hutton, C. F. (1959), "Vertebral arteriography by percutaneous brachial artery catheterisation", *Brit. J. Radiol.*, **32**, 114.

Schechter, M. M. (1961), "Total vertebrobasilar arteriography using a single vertebral puncture technique", *J. Neurosurg.*, **18**, 74.

Seldinger, S. I. (1953), "Catheter replacement of the needle in percutaneous arteriography. A new technique", *Acta radiol., Stockh.*, **39**, 368.

Shands, A. R. Jr. and Bundens, W. D. (1956), "Congenital deformities of the spine; an analysis of the spines of 700 children", *Bull. Hosp. Jt. Dis.*, **17**, 110.

Shapiro, R. (1962), "Myelography", Year book medical publishers, Chicago.

Sharp., J., Purser, D. W. and Lawrence, J. S. (1958), "Rheumatoid arthritis of the cervical spine in the adult", *Ann. rheum. Dis.*, **17**, 303.

Shimidzu, K. (1937), "Beiträge zur Arteriographie des Gehirns—einfache percutane Methode", *Arch. klin. Chir.*, **188**, 295.

Still, G. F. (1897), "On a form of chronic joint disease in children", *Med.-chir. Trans.*, **80**, 47.

Sugar, O., Holden, L. B. and Powell, C. B. (1949), "Vertebral angiography", *Amer. J. Roentgenol.*, **61**, 166.

Tatelman, M. and Sheehan, S. (1962), "Total vertebral-basilar arteriography via transbrachial catheterisation", *Radiology*, **78**, 919.

Thomas, A. E. (1955), "Chronic arthritis after recurrent rheumatic fever", *Ann. rheum. Dis.*, **14**, 259.

Tishler, J. and Martel, W. (1965), "Dislocation of the atlas in mongolism", *Radiology*, **84**, 904.

Wolf, B. S., Khilnani, M. and Malis, L. (1956), "The sagittal diameter of the bony cervical spinal canal and its significance in cervical spondylosis", *J. Mt. Sinai Hosp.*, **23**, 283.

Ziff, M., Contreras, V. and McEwen, C. (1956), "Spondylitis in post-pubertal patients with rheumatoid arthritis of juvenile onset", *Ann. rheum. Dis.*, **17**, 40.

Chapter VI

Differential Diagnosis

MARCIA WILKINSON

Cervical spondylosis is a common cause of both root and cord signs and diagnostic difficulty may arise in relation to cervical spondylosis in one of three ways. Firstly cervical spondylosis may be present but is not the cause of symptoms of which the patient complains. Secondly cervical spondylosis is present in association with an independent disorder of the nervous system and both contribute to the clinical picture. Thirdly the radiological changes in the cervical spine, although simulating spondylosis, are due to some other disorder which is the cause of the neurological symptoms.

(1) CERVICAL SPONDYLOSIS IS PRESENT BUT IS NOT THE CAUSE OF THE SYMPTOMS

In some patients the radiological changes of cervical spondylosis are present but clinical symptoms and signs are due to another cause. These symptoms and signs may be due to a neuropathy, a radiculopathy or a myelopathy or to a combination of any of these.

(a) THE SYMPTOMS SIMULATE A RADICULOPATHY

(i) The median nerve

Compression of the median nerve in the carpal tunnel (the carpal tunnel syndrome). In this syndrome the common complaints are pain and paraesthesiae in the thumb, index and middle finger with sensory loss of median distribution, that is to say impaired sensation on the palmar surface of the thumb, index and middle and radial side of the ring fingers and over the distal phalanx of the same digits associated with weakness and wasting of the muscles of the thenar eminence. In the early stages of a median nerve lesion the pain and paraesthesiae characteristically develop either during the night or are present on waking in the morning. This gives a picture very similar to that of a C6–7 root lesion and a likely source of confusion is that in the carpal tunnel syndrome pain may spread above the wrist and even up to the elbow. The main difference between the sensory disturbance is that in a root lesion the sensory loss is over the back of the digits as well as the front whereas in a lesion of the median nerve it is only on the anterior aspect and on the back of the terminal phalanx of the digits. In the carpal tunnel syndrome the reflexes in the upper limb are usually normal whereas in cervical radiculopathy one or more is usually diminished. In cases of doubt, measurement of nerve conduction velocities is a valuable way of establishing whether or not there is a lesion of the median nerve. One further difficulty arises because the association of carpal tunnel syndrome with cervical spondylosis is common and both may be contributing to the symptoms.

(ii) The ulnar nerve—pressure neuritis of the ulnar nerve

The ulnar nerve is derived from the 8th cervical and 1st thoracic roots. A lesion of the ulnar nerve causes pain and paraesthesiae referred to the little finger and ulnar side of the ring finger with sensory loss of similar distribution and weakness and wasting of the muscles innervated by the nerve particularly of the small muscles of the hand but sparing the lateral part of the thenar eminence. The anatomical distribution of the muscle wasting and sensory loss in an ulnar nerve lesion is distinctive and very unlike that found in radiculopathy due to cervical spondylosis as it is very uncommon for the C8–T1 roots to be involved on their own in cervical spondylosis (see Table 3.1). The ulnar nerve is usually compressed at or about the elbow and motor nerve conduction times may be valuable in localising the lesion, estimating its severity and assessing recovery. There may be thickening or tenderness of the nerve as it passes behind the elbow.

(iii) The costo-clavicular syndrome

This term covers symptoms of a wide range of abnormalities some of which are congenital, the lesion usually being at the level of the thoracic inlet. When such a lesion causes pain in the arm the pain may wrongly be attributed to co-existing cervical spondylosis. However the symptoms in a costo-clavicular syndrome are usually due to pressure upon the inner cord of the brachial plexus which causes wasting of the small muscles of the hand and impairment of cutaneous sensibility on the two ulnar fingers, the ulnar side of the hand and the lower half of the inner aspect of the forearm. This distribution of symptoms and signs is practically unknown as a result of a radiculopathy due to cervical spondylosis and confusion is most likely to occur when there is no X-ray evidence of the abnormality causing the pressure on the inner cord of the plexus. That is to say when there is a cervical rib present this error of diagnosis is unlikely but if there is a fibrous band of the scalenus anterior causing the pressure the differential diagnosis is much more difficult. Symptoms of the costo-clavicular syndrome are particularly likely to be due to traction on the arm (e.g. from carrying of heavy loads) or from loss of tone in the shoulder muscles.

(iv) Neuralgic amyotrophy

This syndrome is characterised by a period of severe pain in one arm of root distribution, followed after a day or two by the development of severe weakness of the muscles usually innervated by one or two roots, the pain subsiding as the weakness develops. Some cases occur spontaneously while others follow injections or inoculations. Unlike the radiculopathy of cervical spondylosis the pain is not greatly affected by movements of the neck. Although such patients may have radiological evidence of cervical spondylosis the very acute onset and severe muscle weakness are unlike the usual findings in cervical spondylosis unless there has been a recent severe injury to the neck.

(v) Cardiac pain

Pain extending down the left arm is a common symptom of cardiac ischaemia and, as it sometimes appears to be of root distribution, may be confused with the radicular pain of cervical spondylosis, especially if there are radiological changes of spondylosis present. In these patients the diagnosis depends on the history, examination and abnormal findings in the electrocardiograph. It is important that the correct diagnosis should be made because it is undesirable that patients with coronary disease should be given active exercises and equally undesirable that patients with root pain should be treated as cardiac invalids.

(b) Cervical spondylosis is present together with symptoms which simulate a cervical myelopathy but are due to some other cause

Occasionally a spinal tumour may co-exist with cervical spondylosis and there may be diagnostic difficulties when it involves the spinal cord at the cervical level. Here the diagnosis can usually be made by myelography and the cerebro-spinal fluid protein is usually higher when a spinal cord neoplasm is present than in spondylosis.

The co-existence of cervical spondylosis and motor neurone disease may cause difficulty, because exceptionally myelopathy due to cervical spondylosis may cause only motor symptoms, namely, muscular wasting, weakness and fasciculation in the upper limbs and spastic weakness of the lower limbs, a clinical picture much resembling that of motor neurone disease. However, the course of such a myelopathy usually extends over years and its progress is much slower than that of motor neurone disease in which muscular wasting is more actively progressive and the accompanying fasciculation much more coarse, widespread and continuous. Moreover, one does not see in cervical spondylosis the cold, cyanosed, wasted hands characteristic of the advanced stages of motor neurone disease and fasciculation in cervical spondylosis is usually limited to one segment. Finally, of course, the presence of any bulbar symptons would clinch the diagnosis in favour of motor neurone disease and the presence of sensory symptoms and signs of root distribution would be much in favour of a diagnosis of cervical spondylosis.

Occasionally there may be difficulty in distinguishing intracranial lesions from those caused by cervical spondylosis. Cerebro-vascular disease may be a source of error especially when the onset of symptoms is insidious and the motor and sensory signs are bilateral. This is most likely to occur when there is ischaemia of the brain stem or cervical cord. Intracranial tumours rarely cause difficulty but in some posterior fossa tumours, when there is no papilloedema, and there are signs of bilateral pyramidal lesions and the headache is occipital, the symptoms may wrongly be attributed to cervical spondylosis.

Cervical spondylosis may give rise to vertigo, especially on lateral rotation or extension of the neck, due to vertebrobasilar insufficiency. Diagnostic difficulties may arise when cervical spondylosis co-exists with vertigo due to another cause. Ménière's syndrome should be readily recognised by its paroxysmal character and the associated deafness and tinnitus, and characteristic findings on audiometric and vestibular investigation. The same applies to an acoustic neuroma which, in addition to focal neurological signs, is associated with characteristic changes in the cerebrospinal fluid and radiological evidence of erosion of the internal auditory meatus. Perhaps the greatest difficulty is likely to arise when benign positional vertigo occurs in a patient who also has cervical spondylosis. The characteristic response of such patients to head rotation in the standard test is usually pathognomonic but in the last resort, when vertigo is caused by head rotation, the only way to decide whether this is due to rotation of the head on the neck or change of position of the labyrinth in space is to compare the effects of rotating the head on the neck with rotation of the whole patient in an appropriate frame. Caloric tests may assist diagnosis.

Psychogenic pain may affect any part of the body and when it involves one upper limb in a patient who has cervical spondylosis, the latter may be wrongly regarded as the cause of the pain. The emotional attitude of the patient in such cases often provides a clue, together with the fact that other symptoms and signs characteristic of a radiculopathy are absent.

(2) CERVICAL SPONDYLOSIS IS PRESENT AND IS PARTIALLY RESPONSIBLE FOR THE SYMPTOMS IN ASSOCIATION WITH ANOTHER DISORDER

(a) Multiple sclerosis

The association of cervical spondylosis and multiple sclerosis was described by Brain and Wilkinson (1957). In such cases, the resulting clinical picture may be atypical of either. There may be no symptoms or signs of multiple sclerosis above the level of the foramen magnum, and the spinal cord lesion may follow the steadily progressive course not uncommonly seen in multiple sclerosis in middle-aged patients and resembling that of cervical myelopathy. However there are helpful distinguishing features. In particular, the occurrence of dysaesthesiae in one or both lower limbs, spreading up to involve the lower part of the trunk is suggestive of multiple sclerosis, as are loss of the abdominal reflexes and the early occurrence of sphincter disturbance, both of which occur late, if at all, in the uncomplicated myelopathy of cervical spondylosis. Examination of the cerebrospinal fluid may be helpful, since the presence of an excess of cells and an abnormal colloidal gold curve in such circumstances is pathognomonic of multiple sclerosis.

(b) Subacute combined degeneration and malabsorption syndromes

The co-existence of these may also lead to difficulties, since the clinical picture may easily be attributed purely to the cervical spondylosis if the evidence of neuropathy in the lower limbs is slight and the necessary investigations to establish the presence of vitamin B12 or folic acid deficiency are not carried out. On the other hand, the patient may be known to have vitamin B12 deficiency and the neurological symptoms be attributed entirely to that, whereas X-rays of the cervical spine will demonstrate the presence of the spondylosis which may be contributing to the symptoms by further damaging an already abnormal spinal cord.

(c) Diabetes mellitus

When a patient suffers from both cervical spondylosis and diabetes mellitus, the resulting neurological disorder, especially in the upper limbs, may be due both to the cervical spondylosis and a diabetic neuropathy. Such patients may have wasting of the small muscles of the hands, together with distal sensory loss in the upper limbs with some evidence of neuropathy in the lower limbs, and with or without the signs of a myelopathy due to the cervical spondylosis.

(d) Vascular disease

As mentioned above, cervical spondylosis frequently co-exists with atheroma involving the vertebral and basilar arteries. In such cases, the cervical spondylosis may add to the embarrassment of the vertebro-basilar circulation. On the other hand, it is important to remember that this is not necessarily the case and the atheroma of the vertebro-basilar system may be substantially unaffected by co-existing cervical spondylosis.

(3) CERVICAL SPONDYLOSIS IS NOT PRESENT BUT IS SIMULATED BY OTHER X-RAY ABNORMALITIES OF THE CERVICAL SPINE

The various conditions which may occur in the cervical spine and in some ways simulate the radiological changes seen in cervical spondylosis have already been discussed in Chapter V and only one or two further points need to be mentioned here. Rheumatoid arthritis of the cervical spine may itself cause a radiculopathy and a myelopathy resembling those due to cervical spondylosis. The symptoms and signs are very similar and here the diagnosis would depend on the other features of rheumatoid arthritis being found, including the joint changes, raised sedimentation rate, positive latex tests, etc. Cervical arthropathy may occur in syringomyelia, tabes dorsalis or diabetes mellitus. In syringomyelia (Brain and Wilkinson, 1958) cervical arthropathy may occur but the characteristic clinical picture of syringomyelia, with a dissociated sensory loss does not resemble the myelopathy of cervical spondylosis. However the symptoms of syringomyelia may be made worse by the effects of the arthropathy on the abnormal spinal cord. Arthropathy of the cervical spine occurring in tabes dorsalis may cause a radiculopathy which in many ways is very similar to that found in spondylosis but once again the characteristic clinical features of tabes should establish the correct diagnosis. Cervical arthropathy may also occur in diabetes but once again the diagnosis depends on the general clinical picture. The radiological abnormalities of the cervical spine found in secondary carcinoma, gout, fluorosis and steroid therapy are fully discussed in Chapter V.

References

Brain, W. R. and Wilkinson, M. (1957), *Brain*, **80**, 456.
Brain, W. R. and Wilkinson, M. (1958), *Brain*, **81**, 275.

Chapter VII

Medical Treatment

G. O. Storey

Introduction

Opinion is divided as to which of the many treatments used for cervical spondylosis is the most satisfactory, but whichever form is adopted careful clinical and radiological assessment is essential before planning teatment and it is also particularly important to exclude other possible causes of pain in the neck and upper limbs. In any treatment the following must be taken into consideration; severity of symptoms, the presence or absence of neurological signs and the severity of the radiological changes in the cervical spine.

Medical treatment is, as a rule, directed to relief of the symptoms of pain and stiffness in the neck and arms, and the different forms of treatment available are reviewed here, together with suggestions for dealing with the various clinical syndromes encountered in conjunction with cervical spondylosis. Special consideration is given to cases with evidence of cord involvement (myelopathy) and also to those in which the vertebral arteries are involved (the vertebrobasilar syndrome).

Bed Rest and Drugs

Bed rest is used mainly in severe acute cases, in chronic cases where there is an acute exacerbation of symptoms and in patients in whom ambulant treatment has failed. It has also been recommended as an initial treatment in cervical spondylosis with myelopathy (Brain and Wilkinson, 1967).

The patient should lie flat in bed with only one pillow and with the head in the most comfortable position, this being maintained with sandbags. As it is important to relieve pain and keep the patient still, adequate analgesics must be given. Salicylates or paracetamol given regularly are usually sufficient but occasionally the pain is so severe that dihydrocodeine (DF118) or physeptone may be necessary.

Indomethacin 25 mg or Phenylbutazone 100 mg eight hourly are sometimes effective in relieving pain but it is not clear why some patients respond to these drugs while others obtain no benefit from them. Morphine derivatives are not to be recommended for chronic cases but may be necessary initially in acute traumatic cases. Hypnotics may be necessary to allay restlessness and Diazepam (Valium) has been used in cases when muscle tension is thought to be an additional cause of symptoms (Bain, 1964). With complete bed rest and regular analgesics the symptoms usually subside within 3–7 days. When the patient is free from pain active exercises may be started and the patient allowed up after a minimum of 2 weeks in bed. In the early stages a soft collar may be used and later a firmer one may be necessary.

Collars

Most authors recommend the use of collars as part of the treatment of cervical spondylosis. Bradshaw (1957) considers them to be the mainstay of treatment and Cyriax (1962) recommends a collar to maintain improvement after manipulation. It has been suggested (Liversedge *et al.*, 1953) that cervical spondylosis produces its effects by direct pressure of osteophytes on the nerve roots and cord, this pressure may be constant or intermittent and may cause interference with the blood supply. A further factor in the causation of acute symptoms may be swelling of the soft tissues of the intervertebral articulations (Dimsdale, 1954). It therefore seems that in cervical spondylosis limitation of neck movement is likely to be helpful and collars are used to achieve this end.

Many different types of collar are available, ranging from those which immobilise the cervical spine to those intended to provide temporary support and limit excessive movement. It is not possible to describe all the varieties of collar but some of the main types can be mentioned.

The Minerva Collar

This encloses the head excluding the face and extends down to the chest wall. This produces good immobilisation of the neck, and is particularly recommended as conservative treatment in cases of cervical spondylosis with myelopathy (Campbell and Phillips, 1960); these writers suggest that a minerva collar should be worn for 3 months. These collars are very uncomfortable, but as the cord symptoms may to some extent be reversed, it is considered that the discomfort should be tolerated.

Polythene Semi-Minerva Collars

These provide a fair amount of immobilisation and can be made to measure and are also lighter to wear than plaster collars, and can be taken off and washed. Bradshaw (1957) found that 11 out of 13 patients with root pain had relief of symptoms in a matter of weeks after wearing a polythene collar and sometimes there was improvement in patients with a myelopathy. On the whole those with generalised spondylosis did less well than those with focal spondylosis. Cyriax (1962) considered that a perspex collar was less obvious and therefore preferable, but this material may be too rigid to be comfortable.

A polythene collar, suitably padded, is well tolerated and is probably the best for long-term use, though adequate ventilation is important as these collars tend to become hot. Liversedge, Hutchinson and Lyons (1953) recommend a leather collar when there is lower motor neurone involvement and consider it should be worn continuously for 3 months and then intermittently. Initially it should be worn at night as well as by day.

Cervical Brace

This type of collar consists of a chin cup and occipital plate with adjustable metal supports resting on a chest piece. The angle of flexion can be adjusted to avoid pressure round the neck. This type of collar is rather cumbersome and in practice does not stand up to mechanical stresses and strains and therefore is not often found to be satisfactory.

The Thomas Collar

There are many variations of this type of collar which is small and light and provides some support for the neck and limits excessive movement. These collars may be made of plastic, sorbo, foam, felt or rubber, these last being inflatable, and are usually fastened by straps and buckles or velcro fasteners. The optimum position of the spine is in slight flexion with the chin indrawn and one of the difficulties of this type of collar is that they tend to extend the neck. This is undesirable as the patient cannot then easily see his feet and is liable to trip. The collars made from these materials are rather hot and uncomfortable to wear but simple collars of this type are very suitable for less severe cases; there is little to choose between the various patterns.

The Lewin Collar

This consists of a length of felt which can be wrapped round the neck and fastened with tape. It may be rather hot but is soft and suitable for night wear.

The Victoria Collar

This is composed of a malleable metal frame with a rubber cover which can be moulded to fit the neck. This type of collar is made commercially and the correct size must be selected for the patient.

Temporary Collars

Can be made on the spot by cutting out lengths of felt, plastic foam or foam rubber, or even newspaper and tying them in position round the neck. New plastic materials can also be used for making temporary collars. Some of these materials, e.g. Prenol and Plastazote, become malleable when heated to a given temperature and can be moulded to fit the patient's neck thus providing an immediate firm support. Prenol and Plastazote have the additional advantage that they are poor conductors of heat and can therefore be moulded directly on to the neck without burning the skin, and they do not require a lining. Polythene can be used in a similar way but will become hot and requires a foam insulator. Strips of velcro can be used as fastening material. Ideally a collar should be high at the back with a front fastening as this maintains the correct position of the neck and can be easily taken off and put on (Fig. 7.1).

Before providing a collar it is essential to assess the degree of disability, and the type of collar selected should depend on the degree of immobilisation required. Sorbo rubber, felt or foam collars will restrict gross movement—while plaster and plastic collars will give better immobilisation. Any collar should fit well and maintain the neck in the most comfortable position. In spite of this many people, particularly men, dislike wearing collars (Steinberg and Mason, 1959). Other patients however, particularly women, seem to become addicted to wearing them and it is difficult to persuade them to leave them off. It is probably as well to advise leaving the collar off after about

3 months because otherwise weakness and wasting of the neck muscles may occur. After the acute painful stage is over it is sometimes helpful to give active exercises in conjunction with the wearing of a collar.

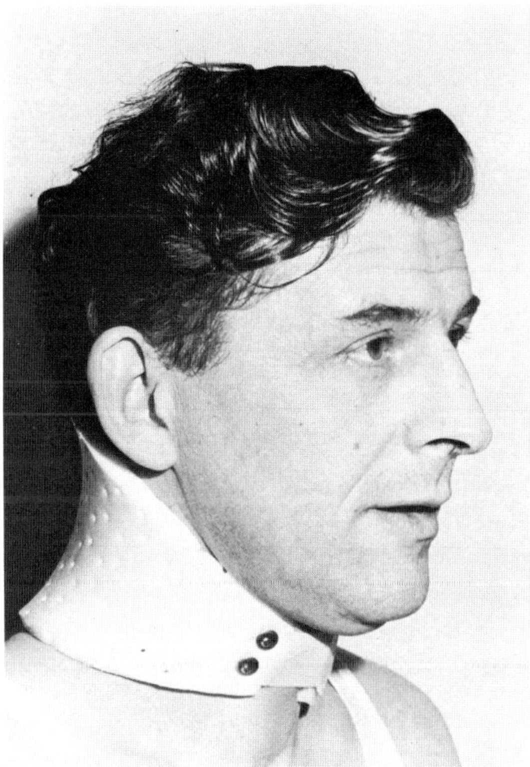

Fig. 7.1 Temporary collar made of Plastazote, higher at the back and with front fastening

TRACTION

This may be either continuous or intermittent.

Continuous Traction

This type of traction is used in the more severe acute cases and when the symptoms of root compression are marked. Various methods of fixing the head are used. The most efficient is ice-tong calipers in the skull but a halo head band or a Sayers sling with a chin strap may be used.

Traction is usually only used when bed rest alone has failed because if bed rest and immobilisation of the spine are strictly enforced it will seldom be necessary to use continuous traction. Some patients cannot tolerate traction and a few are made worse by it. In any case analgesics and hypnotics must be used in sufficient doses to prevent restlessness. Nursing may also be a problem and some patients have difficulty in micturition when immobilised. It is sometimes useful to set up the traction apparatus, but use only 5 lb in weight; this will have the effect of keeping the patient still in bed while any unpleasant effects of traction are avoided. However, stronger traction may be considered necessary when bed rest alone has failed and Crisp (1960) believes it can shorten the period of bed rest.

Methods of Traction

Ice-tong calipers or a halo head band allow more freedom of the mouth for feeding and prevent strain on the tempero-mandibular joints, damage to which has been reported after the use of a head halter with chin strap (Franks, 1964). There is some difference in opinion as to the correct direction of pull. Wareham and Farrow (1960) believe that the most comfortable position should be found and traction exerted in this direction, in which case, as the muscle spasm improves, the head gradually assumes a neutral position. Cyriax (1965) considers that the head should be in extension while Christie (1965) considered that slight flexion was the best position. About 10 lb weight is attached to a cord over a pulley and the head of the bed raised to increase the pull and prevent the trunk sliding up. The weight may be increased to 20 lb according to muscular development or may be varied during the day. Cyriax recommends 10–12 lb by day and 5–8 lb at night. There is no evidence that weights of this range will cause distraction of the vertebrae and Yates, Goodman and Wilson (1966) state that a force of 30–60 lb is required to do this. However, no authors recommend weights of this magnitude in continuous traction and many believe that traction used in this way only ensures complete immobilisation. It is claimed that symptoms of brachial neuralgia will be relieved within a few days and when this has been achieved the amount of traction can be gradually reduced, leaving it off for half-hour periods to begin with. When the traction has been stopped a collar should be provided and the patient allowed up; he should also be encouraged to do active exercises.

In acute traumatic lesions of the cervical spine with root compression, if traction provides no relief after 2 weeks, surgery should be considered (Brain and Wilkinson, 1967). Although some patients find traction unpleasant, there are few reports of serious adverse effects of traction but Wilkinson (1964) reported a patient who developed a hemianopic field defect after traction. This form of treatment is unsuitable for patients with gross radiological changes in the cervical spine because of the danger of cord compression or pressure on the vertebral arteries. Extending the spine may narrow the saggittal (AP) diameter of the spinal canal by 2 mm thus reducing the diameter below the critical level of 11 mm.

Intermittent traction

This may be applied manually or mechanically by pulley and weight with a head halter.

Manual traction may be applied directly to the head, one hand holding the occiput and the other placed under the chin. In this way the direction of pull can be easily adjusted, but it is emphasised that training is necessary before attempting this. Cyriax (1962) recommends this type of traction in some cases as a preliminary to manipulation and claims that he can exert a force of up to 300 lb. However traction of this magnitude will not usually be applied and some physicians use manual traction only to assess the suitability of the patient for a course of traction. Manual traction may also be applied using a sling and head halter, the traction being applied to the separating bar.

Mechanical traction is by head halter or pulley and weight. Heat and gentle mobilising exercises are sometimes used as a preliminary and traction is applied with the patient lying on a plinth. The direction of pull is selected as in continuous traction usually in the most comfortable position. A weight of between 15–25 lb is generally used and traction applied for 15–20 minutes, the treatment being repeated daily if necessary. Crisp (1960) advises 25–40 lb for 20–30 minutes with the head at an angle of 35–40° to the horizontal and, when improvement occurs, the use of manual traction or gentle manipulation.

Relief of root pain often occurs immediately traction is applied even though the weight used is insufficient to cause any separation of vertebrae but is likely to recur when traction is relaxed sometimes with an increase of pain. In a few patients the pain is aggravated by traction. It is thought that the immediate relief of pain is due to the overcoming of muscular spasm.

Head suspension is another form of mechanical traction which may be applied and for this the patient is placed in a sitting position so that the weight of the body acts as the distracting force when the buttocks are raised off the seat for 1–5 minutes (Cyriax, 1965). However the distracting force is considerable and this form of traction is not considered suitable for older patients and those suffering from obesity, severe spondylosis or hypertension. A Kuhlmann apparatus has also been used to apply traction and can be used in the home. Air pressure is used as the distracting force and the amount measured on a manometer.

The disadvantages and dangers of traction have already been discussed and until recently there have been few efforts made to assess its therapeutic value. Steinberg and Mason (1959) in a small pilot study found that longitudinal traction given either manually or mechanically by means of a Sayers sling or by a Kuhlmann apparatus with a 15 lb pull for 15 minutes, had no advantage over a felt collar or neck and shoulder girdle exercises. The British Association of Physical Medicine trial (1966) used traction for 20 minutes with the head in the most comfortable position. They found that while this might temporarily relieve symptoms at the time of application and for several hours afterwards, it did not affect the rate of recovery, and they concluded that the indications for traction as out-patient treatment were few, except in cases of severe pain unrelieved by simpler methods of treatment.

Active exercise therapy has been used in most regimes of treatment, the exercises falling into the following three groups:

1. Neck mobilising exercises.
2. Shoulder raising exercises.
3. Muscle strengthening exercises.

Steinberg and Mason (1959) have listed some of these but most centres adopt their own variations and indeed to avoid monotony, exercises should be varied. The exercises may be given individually or in groups.

1. Neck mobilising exercises

These have been used as a preliminary to traction (B.A.P.M. 1966), and have been used following manipulation to maintain mobility.

2. Shoulder raising exercises

These exercises aim to elevate the shoulder girdle thus relieving drag on the nerve roots and any symptoms resulting from thoracic inlet pressure and can be combined with the use of a collar. The following are some typical examples.

(a) Arm raising sideways and upwards over head.
(b) Arms bend; arms stretching upwards.
(c) Shoulder shrugging.
(d) Arm raising forwards and upwards over head.
(e) Arms bend, finger-tips touching. Shoulder and elbows circling backwards.
(f) Arms raising sideways to 90°, arms pressing backwards.

3. Muscle strengthening exercises

To achieve an increase in muscle power some resistance must be introduced and the exercises listed above may be carried out with varying weights held in the hands or placed on the shoulders. A basket ball may be used in group therapy, the patients catching and throwing with the arms above the head. These exercises will help in strengthening the shoulder girdle muscles. The use of progressive exercises has been described by Colson (1958) and Gardiner (1957). Strengthening exercises for the neck muscles are more difficult to carry out as any resistance is likely to place a strain on the cervical spine. However it is advantageous to try and strengthen these muscles as they are the ones which become weakened by wearing a collar. It has been claimed that the use of *Proprioceptive neuromuscular facilitation* (P.N.F.) may overcome this difficulty and that maximum contractions of the neck muscles can be obtained using only minimal resistance. The techniques of this type of treatment can be found in specialised books. Their use is time-consuming and special training is required to carry them out.

Head positioning. In some cases symptoms can be relieved if the head is placed in a particular position (Brewerton, 1964). This is the position of maximum comfort in which traction may be applied (Wareham and Farrow, 1960; Brain and Wilkinson, 1967). However, even if the head is maintained in this position for 20 minutes without traction, relief of symptoms will occur. In their trial the British Association of Physical

Medicine (1966) used this method followed by wearing of a collar and found it as effective as the other forms of treatment.

Posture instructions. All patients should be instructed in correct positioning of the head both during the day and in bed, and told to avoid holding it awkwardly when reading, driving and watching television. Sudden jerks and movements of the neck should be avoided and the provision of a headrest in the car may help. The head should be carried at all times in its optimum position of slight flexion with the chin indrawn (Brain and Wilkinson, 1967).

Massage. This is not often used now in the treatment of cervical spondylosis. However, painful areas of muscle spasm in the muscles may be relieved by massage.

Injection of local anaesthetic or hydrocortisone into painful areas may give relief of pain and spasm and improvement in cervical movement (Lishman and Ritchie Russell, 1961).

Heat in the form of radiant heat or short-wave diathermy will also help to relieve muscle spasm and is used as an adjuvant to treatment by manipulation, traction, exercises and massage.

Other Forms of Treatment

Lishman and Ritchie Russell (1961) point out that there is often an overlap in the various causes of pain in the upper limb and thus inlet and carpal tunnel syndromes often produce very similar clinical pictures to those found in cervical spondylosis. They suggest the use of a small sorbo-rubber collar to limit excessive movement of the neck but advise resting the arm in a sling, with local injections of procaine round the scapula. They avoid all active forms of physiotherapy. If this is unsuccessful treatment must be considered at other sites in the arm. The recent description of other entrapment syndromes has suggested further possible sites to which treatment may be directed.

Stiff shoulder. This condition and its treatment is discussed later.

Tennis elbow. Occasionally symptoms of this condition are associated with root pain due to cervical spondylosis. Local injection of hydrocortisone to the tender point should be used in addition to other forms of treatment.

Manipulation. The effectiveness of manipulation of the cervical spine cannot be assessed since there are no figures available for comparison with other methods, and this has led to conflicting views on its effectiveness and dangers. Some patients believe that manipulation has cured their pain whilst others consider that they were made worse by it.

The techniques of manipulation will not be described here as they may be found elsewhere (Crisp, 1960; Maitland, 1964; Cyriax, 1965). Theoretically if the exact nature of the spinal displacement, if any, can be diagnosed, and replaced by manipulation without endangering the nervous system, then this would be a desirable form of treatment (Richardson, 1957). Crisp (1960) believes that disturbances in the zygapophyseal joints would be particularly amenable to manipulation and would respond to this treatment, as might other minor displacements. Unfortunately there is as yet no certain way of diagnosing the type of disturbance which causes symptoms in a particular case and it seems unlikely from a study of the anatomy of the cervical spine that much actual displacement of the bony structures can occur except after major injury. Although those who practice manipulation have sought to establish the criteria and the contra-indications for its use, the pathological concepts put forward, e.g. "annular" lesion, "pulp" protrusions, etc., seek to describe a symptom complex and do not have the support of morbid anatomy. It seems probable that the cause of the symptoms is more complex than is at present realised. Christie (1965) states that "annular" lesions respond well to manipulation, "pulp" protrusions do not, while primary posterolateral protrusions respond better to traction. He also states that the presence of motor weakness and reflex changes in the upper limbs are not amenable to manipulation and the occurrence of any myelopathic signs in the lower limbs contra-indicates manipulation. Cyriax (1965) agrees that any evidence of a myelopathic lesion is a contra-indication to manipulation and considers that if there is an increase in pain in the arm during manipulation the treatment should be abandoned. He also believes that "pulp" protrusion does not respond well to this form of treatment. In certain cases he believes manipulation should be preceded by traction, namely when there is considerable spinal deformity, and paraesthesiae in the legs and arms. All authors are agreed that before manipulation is undertaken, careful clinical and radiological examination must be carried out to exclude possible congenital abnormality and other lesions; also that only those who have had careful instruction and experience should carry out these manouvres.

Nevertheless sometimes disasters do occur, and severe neurological complications and death have been described by Pratt, Thomas and Berger (1947), Kunkle *et al.* (1952), Ford and Clark (1959), Green and Joynt (1959), Smith and Estridge (1962). These complications have usually resulted from vascular disturbances of the vertebral arteries. These arteries appear to be particularly susceptible at the level of the atlas where they enter the skull. Rotation and hyperextension are regarded as the dangerous movements (Smith and Estridge, 1962). The possible causes of disasters have been summarised as follows (Green and Joynt, 1959):

1. Violent manipulation.
2. Abnormal bony structures, congenital and degenerative.
3. Atherosclerosis.
4. Abnormal vascular patterns.

These conditions cannot always be anticipated and it has been noted that many of the fatalities have occurred in patients in their thirties in whom no gross abnormalities could be demonstrated at post-mortem. However the number of recorded fatalities is not large and Cyriax (1962) believes they have been over-emphasised. Kersley (1952) points a further danger, i.e. that spontaneous subluxation of cervical vertebrae may occur in the presence of tonsillar or pharyngeal sepsis. Smith and Estridge (1962) suggest that accidents may be avoided if the head is first placed in a rotated and hyper-extended position and if this induces any vertigo, faintness or nausea, manipulation is not attempted. Brewerton (1964) suggests that some gentle oscillation at the extremes of the range of movement may avoid the dangers of the forceful movements which often form part of the usual procedure. Manipulation therefore remains a controversial treatment and even if it relieves symptoms, some people have a clinical impression that relapse is more likely, and this would not be surprising since supporting ligaments may well be damaged. Indeed Maitland (1964) states that any vigorous manipulation must have traumatic effects. It seems better, therefore, in view of the uncertainty of its effects and the possible dangers, to avoid this treatment particularly when simpler and safer measures are so often effective.

Conclusions

In view of the foregoing, it is possible to recommend the following lines of treatment.

1. Acute severe syndromes

These are best treated by bed rest with immobilisation of the head between sandbags with sufficient analgesia to relieve pain and control restlessness. Only in rare cases where this fails and when there is severe brachial neuralgia need continuous traction be considered. If continuous traction fails after 2 weeks, then surgery must be considered. This is more likely to be successful if there is evidence of a localised lesion; the presence of diffuse changes in the cervical spine diminish the likelihood of successful surgery. The possibility of some other lesion being present must be considered if immobilisation of the neck and traction fail and this is another reason for surgery at this stage.

2. Less severe syndromes

Assessment of the various forms of treatment available has not been often attempted. Steinberg and Mason (1959) in their pilot study compared (1) heat, massage and traction, (2) felt collar, (3) neck and shoulder girdle exercises. Although their numbers were small they considered that a supporting collar produced the highest improvement rate. The British Association of Physical Medicine (1966) carried out a multicentre trial and compared (1) traction and a collar, (2) positioning of the head, (3) collar alone, (4) placebo treatment. They found that the rate of improvement was approximately the same in all the treatment groups even though traction might produce some temporary relief of root pressure symptoms and some patients were more comfortable in a collar. These findings suggest that the symptoms of cervical spondylosis run a self-limiting course which is not modified by medical treatment. Those treatments which are least likely to cause side effects and most likely to relieve pain should therefore be adopted. Sufficient analgesics should be given and in the milder cases, some simple form of physiotherapy such as heat and shoulder-raising exercises with head positioning and instruction on head posture. This instruction may be combined with injections of local anaesthetic into painful areas of muscle.

With more severe cases a collar, to be worn day and night, should be the mainstay of treatment and this may be combined with the other treatments mentioned above. Traction should only be considered if there are severe root symptoms and other methods have failed. The risks of this should be realised. The effects of manipulation were not investigated in the B.A.P.M. trial (1966) and it would be difficult to incorporate it in a trial since the techniques used by various operators differ so markedly. Those who employ it in the hope of shortening the natural course of the disease must weigh this advantage against the possible dangers. It is not possible to recommend it as a routine method of treatment. The cervical spine is reasonably stable in health but in disease it may be extremely vulnerable. The closeness of vital structures—the spinal cord and the vertebral arteries suggest that distracting or distorting treatments, i.e. traction and manipulation, are best avoided. The possibility that symptoms in the upper limb may be partly or wholly caused by other "entrapment" syndromes should be borne in mind.

Treatment of Cervical Myelopathy

In cervical spondylosis when there are signs of cord compression conservative treatment should be tried first. Medical treatment usually consists of rest in bed and sometimes a collar. If bed rest is tried this should be complete, the patient lying flat for 2–3 weeks. In most patients with spondylotic myelopathy on whom an autopsy has been done, the pathological changes in the cord consist of atrophy, loss of ganglion cells, gliosis and demyelination. It seems unlikely that, once these changes have occurred, any form of treatment will make any difference. Treatment is therefore only likely to be effective if instituted in the early phase of the disorder and before there are irreversible changes. If a patient with cervical spondylosis, who has recently deteriorated, is rested, there is very often an improvement in the symptoms and physical signs, which could be due to a subsidence of oedema. Some patients make a very good functional recovery although most of them are left with residual neurological signs. If, however, there are signs of increasing cord compression operation is likely to have the best results if carried out in the first few months and decision to operate should not be delayed. See Chapter VIII.

The Treatment of Vertebro-basilar Ischaemia

As Hutchinson and Yates (1956) have pointed out, atheroma frequently occurs in patients in whom there is distortion of the vertebral artery by cervical spondylosis. This common association in elderly people of cervical spondylosis and atheroma within the vertebro-basilar circulation is important in relation to treatment. In these people symptoms are often produced by active or passive movements of the head and this suggests that, in certain positions of the head, osteophytes may be compressing one or both vertebral arteries. These patients should be advised to avoid all movements that they know are likely to bring on symptoms, most often turning the head to the right or left, looking upward or bending down. Collars are useful because they limit movement and remind the patient of his disability.

STIFF (FROZEN) SHOULDER

Pain in the shoulder is often a symptom of cervical spondylosis and it has been suggested (Coventry, 1953) that any condition which causes pain in the shoulder may give rise to a stiff shoulder and thus cervical spondylosis must be considered a precipitating factor. The causes of pain in the shoulder are numerous and a consideration of them all is outside the scope of this book. Coventry (1953) gives a list of them and Mattingly (1960) has reviewed the subject. It should be noted that pain in the shoulder may be caused either by lesions which lie in and around the shoulder joint, or by conditions which cause referred pain in the shoulder. These may lie either in or around the cervical spine, or in the thorax, heart and lungs, or above or below the diaphragm.

Other factors which may be important in the causation of the frozen shoulder are immobility and psychological factors. There is a third group in which no associated abnormality can be found, and in these cases the stiff shoulder must be regarded as idiopathic. Trauma is a common cause of a frozen shoulder and injuries to the capsule and associated tendons (rotator cuff lesion, supraspinnatus tendonitis) may all be followed by a limitation of all movements of the joint (frozen shoulder). The condition is rare before the age of 40 so that degenerative changes in the tendons and capsule are also likely to be important. Pathologically the changes found in the capsule are those of the reparative stage of inflammation (Neviaser, 1957) and the terms capsulitis and periarthritis are therefore also used. The association of the frozen shoulder with referred pain is more difficult to explain. Some believe that immobility associated with pain will suffice as an explanation but it seems unlikely that this is the whole truth. Some believe that the shoulder changes result from a reflex sympathetic dystrophy (Steinbrocker *et al.*, 1948). It is postulated that pain stimulae from various sources irritate the neurones in the spinal cord and that a discharge of sympathetic impulses results in changes in the shoulder presumably resulting from vascular effects. Changes may also occur in the hand on the affected side and these appear also to be sympathetic in nature ("shoulder-hand syndrome"). The hand first swells and becomes red, hot and painful and later atrophic changes develop with fibrosis in the palm and Sudek's atrophy. Support for this theory is provided by the fact that relief is sometimes obtained at least temporarily by stellate ganglion block. Cardiac pain is a well documented cause of the stiff shoulder and shoulder-hand syndrome and in this condition afferent impulses must travel via the sympathetic nerve to the central nervous system. In this condition temperature changes in the left arm have been recorded, suggesting that a disturbance of the sympathetic system does in fact occur (Donet and Ferrero, 1951).

The relationship of cervical spondylosis to these changes in the shoulder and hand is of less certainty. Oppenheimer (1938) in a series of cases of swollen hand of sympathetic type correlated these changes with osteoarthritic changes in the cervical spine and believed that involvement of the foramen of C4 was the important lesion. Coventry (1953) reported that there was often a history of stiff neck in patients with a frozen shoulder and considered that irritation of the nerve roots was an important aetiological factor and Brewerton (1969) noted that traction of the cervical spine would sometimes relieve a stiff shoulder. Steinbrocker *et al.* (1948) also considered intraforaminal osteoarthritis to be a cause of reflex dystrophy of the upper limb. On the other hand Cogman (1934) reported that cervical spondylosis caused pain in the shoulder usually without stiffness, and in a series of 67 cases of stiff shoulder Storey (1959) reported that only three cases had clinical evidence of cervical spondylosis (i.e. a stiff neck). Radiological changes of cervical spondylosis are likely to be common in patients with stiff shoulders since these are almost invariably found after the age of 40 when degenerative changes in the cervical spine are common. However pain of root type is a fairly common finding with a stiff shoulder, 21 out of 67 cases (Storey, 1959) and cervical spondylosis may be the cause of both these conditions.

The relationship of herpes zoster to the stiff shoulder and shoulder-hand syndrome is well documented, and cervical spondylosis has been regarded by some as a predisposing cause of herpes zoster. Gramdal (1959) reported a case where the rash involved C5–6 skin area and osteoarthrosis of the intervertebral foramina C4–5 and C5–6 was present. In a case of stiff shoulder, Richardson (1954), the rash involved the 7th and 8th cervical root, an area related to the sympathetic nerve supply to the limb rather than the somatic nerves. Coventry (1953) and Steinbroker *et al.* (1948) also regard herpes as a cause of the frozen shoulder and shoulder-hand syndrome. It seems likely therefore that at least in some cases cervical spondylosis is related to a frozen shoulder and the shoulder-hand syndrome. In the treatment of cervical spondylosis it is better therefore to avoid immobilising the shoulder since it is likely to aggravate stiffness. If a stiff shoulder develops active treatment to encourage movement and heat to the shoulder should be used. In more severe cases the use of local injections of hydrocortisone may be tried but this is only likely to be effective if there is a local lesion in the shoulder (tendonitis, bursitis) rather than when the signs are those of general limitation of movement. In more severe cases a stellate ganglion block may be tried and this may be repeated (Steinbrocker *et al.*, 1953) while prednisone by mouth is also sometimes effective. If pain is severe deep X-ray therapy may be justified. When the painful stage of the disease has passed manipulation has been recommended in order to restore mobility to the shoulder joint. There is evidence that the stiff shoulder is a self-limiting condition so that the natural course of the disease is towards eventual recovery though this may take months or even 1–2 years.

References

Bradshaw, P. (1957), *Quart. J. Med.*, **26**, 771.
Bain, L. S. (1964), *Ann. Phys. Med.*, suppl., p. 3.
Brain, the Lord and Wilkinson, M. (1967), *Cervical Spondylosis*, Heinemann, London.
Brewerton, D. A. (1964), *Proc. roy. Soc. Med.*, **57**, 163.

British Assoc. Phys. Med. (1966), *Brit. med. J.*, **2**, 253.
Campbell, E. G. M. and Phillips, D. G. (1960), *Brit. med. J.*, **2**, 481.
Christie, B. G. B. (1965), *Ann. Phys. Med.*, **8**, 103.
Colson, J. H. C. (1958), *Progressive Exercise Therapy*, Wright, Bristol.
Coventry, M. B. (1953), *J. Amer. med. Assoc.*, **151**, 177.
Crisp, E. J. (1960), *Disc Lesions*, Livingston, London.
Cyriax, J. (1962), *Textbook of Orth. Med.*, Vol. I, Cassell, London.
Cyriax, J. (1965), *Textbook of Orth. Med.*, Vol. II, Cassell, London.
Dimsdale, H. (1954), *Proc. roy. Soc. Med.*, **47**, 54.
Donet, J. P. and Ferrero, C. (1951), *Cardiologia*, **9**, 80.
Ford, F. R. and Clark, D. (1956), *Bull. John Hopk. Hosp.*, **98**, 37.
Franks, A. S. (1964), *Ann. Phys. Med.*, **8**, 38.
Gardiner, M. D. (1957), *The Principles of Exercise Therapy*, Bell, London.
Grandal, H. (1959), *Acta. Rheum. Scand.*, **5**, 157.
Green, D. and Joynt, R. J. (1959), *J. Amer. med. Assoc.*, **1(70)**, 522.
Hutchinson, E. C. and Yates, P. O. (1956), *Brain*, **79**, 319.
Kersley, G. D. (1952), *Ann. Phys. Med.*, **1**, 140.
Kunkle, E. C., Muller, J. C. and Ochem, G. L. (1952), *Ann. Int. Med.*, **36**, 1329.
Lishman, W. A. and Ritchie Russell, W. (1961), *Lancet*, **ii**, 941.
Liversedge, L. A., Hutchinson, E. C. and Lyons, J. B. (1953), *Lancet*, **ii**, 65.
Maitland, G. D. (1964), *Vertebral Manipulation*, Butterworth, London.
Mattingly, S. (1960), *Ann. Phys. Med.*, **5**, 266.
Neviaser, J. S. (1945), *J. Bone Jt. Surg.*, **27**, 211.
Pratt-Thomas, H. R. and Berger, K. E. (1947), *J. Amer. med. Assoc.*, **133**, 600.
Richardson, A. T. (1954), *Ann. Phys. Med.*, **2**, 132.
Richardson, A. T. (1957), *Proc. roy. Soc. Med.*, **50**, 142.
Smith, R. A. and Estridge, M. N. (1962), *J. Amer. Med. Assoc.*, **182**, 528.
Steinberg, V. L. and Mason, R. M. (1959), *Ann. Phys. Med.*, **5**, 37.
Steinbrocker, O., Neustadt, D. H. and Lapin, L. (1953), *J. Amer. med. Ass.*, **153**, 788.
Steinbrocker, O., Spetzenn, N. and Friedman, H. H. (1948), *Ann. Int. Med.*, **29**, 22.
Storey, G. (1959), *Proc. roy. Soc. Med.*, **52**, 759.
Wareham, T. and Farrow, R. (1960), *Lancet*, **ii**, 337.
Wilkinson, M. (1964), *Proc. roy. Soc. Med.*, **57**, 159.
Yates, A., Goodman, H. and Wilson, D. (1966), *Brit. Med. J.*, **1**, 540.

Chapter VIII

Surgical Treatment

L. Symon

While the changes of cervical spondylosis are widespread in patients in advancing years, having been said to be present radiographically in 75 per cent of people aged 50 or over (Kuhlendahl and Kunert, 1954), in the majority of cases the development of spondylosis is not associated with neurological disability. The principal tasks of the surgeon in the assessment of a patient with cervical spondylosis are to assess first how far the spondylosis is related to any neurological dysfunction which the patient suffers, and second, how far surgery may be expected to relieve this.

Pathogenesis

In the planning of any surgical treatment, an appreciation of the pathogenesis of the condition is vital. Two main views have been advanced to explain the involvement of neurological structures by the development of spondylotic changes in the cervical spine and it seems likely that both may have some role. These are dealt with more fully elsewhere in this volume, but may be briefly re-stated here.

In the first, spondylotic changes are considered to cause damage to the vessels of the cervical spine, either within the spinal canal or as they enter upon spinal nerve roots (Mair and Druckman, 1953; Taylor, 1964) with the development of radiculopathy or myelopathy on an ischaemic basis. Permanent changes are found in the cord although they are not necessarily on a vascular basis. Though they are unlikely to be reversed by operation, one may hope to prevent progression.

In the second theory, it is supposed that development of osteophytes, together with the foreshortening of the cervical spine resulting from absorption of the disc spaces with associated buckling in of the ligamentum flavum posteriorly, together result in a diminished available space for the cervical cord which therefore suffers compression and recurrent minor traumata during extension or flexion of the spine. The pathological changes seen in the cervical cord in association with long standing spondylosis would then be produced by trauma and not by vascular occlusion, and they may be prevented by decompression of the cord at an early stage, although it must again be admitted that the changes, once established, can never be reversed.

The probability is that both pathological mechanisms play a part. It is however clear that severe pathology in the spinal cord or in the nerve roots cannot be reversed, and there is much to be said therefore, for undertaking treatment designed to prevent such changes before the disability has progressed too far.

Symptom Complexes Presenting for Surgery

Two main groups of patients present for consideration of surgery.

In the first of these the symptoms are related principally to the roots emerging from the cervical spine, and the condition presents itself with either intermittent neck and arm pain or progressive sensory or motor loss usually in only one arm.

In the second, the condition presents with the development of a slowly progressive, or episodically deteriorating myelopathy involving first the legs and then the arms, and whose principal clinical features are detailed elsewhere within this volume.

In addition to these two main groups, the patients may more rarely present for consideration for operation because of persistent painful stiff neck, or because of a group of symptoms suggesting obstruction of the vertebral artery in the neck by osteophytes laterally placed in the intervertebral foramina. In British clinical practice, both these groups of patients are rare, the first because the painful stiff neck responds in the vast majority of cases to careful and persistent conservative treatment, and the second because this appears to be an extremely rare complication of cervical spondylosis despite the fact that it has been increasingly looked for since the pioneering cases were described (Hardin *et al.*, 1960; Gortvai, 1964; Sheehan *et al.*, 1960; Brain, 1963).

The selection of patients for operation

(a) Operation for radicular symptoms

In the discussion of surgery for arm pain, it is necessary to separate from the discussion the acute painful arm in the relatively young patient, following classically a twist of the neck or the maintenance of the neck for a prolonged period of time in an unnatural position, succeeded within some hours or days by the development of severe radicular pain within the distribution of one nerve root. This is commonly discovered to be due to the lateral protrusion of a soft piece of intervertebral cartilage much analogous to protrusion of a lumbar intervertebral disc. Plain X-rays in such patients frequently show little or no evidence of cervical spondylosis, and the condition is not one properly considered in a chapter devoted to its management. Clear cut radicular pain of sudden onset occurs less commonly in cervical spondylosis, where more chronic painful syndromes with, frequently, evidence of involvement of more than one root, and the development of progressive muscular disability in the arm accompanied by spondylotic changes at a variety of levels, make the assessment of the precise intervertebral foramen involved more difficult. As a rule, the acute episodes of neck and arm pain which occur in association with cervical spondylosis respond particularly well to analgesics and bed rest associated with immobilisation of the cervical spine, perhaps accompanied by gentle traction using a halter type of collar.

Recurrent episodes may be associated with the development of motor disability within the distribution of roots other than those affected by pain and sometimes with a motor distribution suggesting the involvement of more than one root. Provided adequate immobilisation of the neck in a suitable cervical collar has failed to arrest such neurological deterioration, it is reasonable to consider the patient for surgery. In the author's experience surgery for pain alone is rarely necessary in cervical spondylosis.

Adequate clinical investigation supplemented by electrical conduction studies will exclude peripheral nerve disease and the assessment of the case for surgery thereafter depends upon detailed radiology of the cervical spine. This is discussed in Chapter V. Essential films are A.P., lateral and oblique views to show the intervertebral foramina. Osteophytes projecting into the intervertebral foramina are frequently present bilaterally, and it may be difficult to decide why one or two roots should have become particularly involved. Myelography should clarify the situation by demonstrating non-filling of a root sheath laterally towards the intervertebral foramen in one or more roots whose distribution would fit the episodes of pain and the progressive neurological dysfunction. Under these circumstances, surgery is indicated.

(b) Operation for myelopathy

The development of gradually progressive spastic quadriparesis or of episodic deterioration of spastic weakness in the arms and legs, together with progressive unsteadiness of gait related to posterior column loss as detailed in Chapter IV of this volume, is the usual presenting picture suggesting cervical myelopathy. Where changes of cervical spondylosis are present there is a tendency to attribute such myelopathy to spondylosis but it has become all too clear over the years that this attribution cannot be made without fairly rigid criteria being fulfilled.

In this author's view, the demonstration of appreciable narrowing of the cervical canal is an essential prerequisite to the diagnosis of cervical spondylotic myelopathy sufficiently severe to warrant surgery. In this respect it is noteworthy that patients with cervical spondylotic myelopathy generally have a rather narrow cervical canal. This may be demonstrated by measurements from the centre of the vertebral body to the base of the spine of the same vertebra (i.e. away from any possible osteophytic encroachment on the neural canal) (Burrows, 1963; Symon and Lavender, 1967). Thus, Burrows noted that the mean measurement on normal human beings at C5 was 17·7 mm, whereas in a series of patients with spondylotic myelopathy studied by Symon and Lavender, the mean C5 measurement was 13·7 mm. The available diameter of the neural canal is further reduced at the level of the intervertebral discs, by the humped up protrusion of annulus and osteophyte, and measurement of the narrowest distance from a spondylotic bar to the nearest point on the posterior wall of the canal shows even less available space for the cervical cord (Fig. 8.1). Thus Wolf *et al.* (1956) found this measurement to be 10 mm or less in cases showing cord compression and 13 mm or more in cases where no myelopathy occurred. A review of plain films in a series of 48 cases by Symon and Lavender showed this measurement at its narrowest point to be 12 mm or less in 86 per cent of patients with cervical spondylotic myelopathy. As Burrows has pointed out however, measurement on plain film is open to the objection that laterally placed osteophytes which are not associated with cord compression may still narrow the apparent diameter measured in this way and for this reason a more reliable method of assessment of the available diameter of the canal is at myelography. It is important that adequate volumes of Myodil be used, and 6 to 9 cc will generally prove adequate. Frontal and lateral views should be taken with the patient prone and the neck initially in full extension. In this position, any possible block will be at its maximum, and the neck may thereafter be gradually flexed once adequate views of a possible obstruction have been obtained. Cord compression is shown by a complete or partial block in association with a narrow neural canal. The

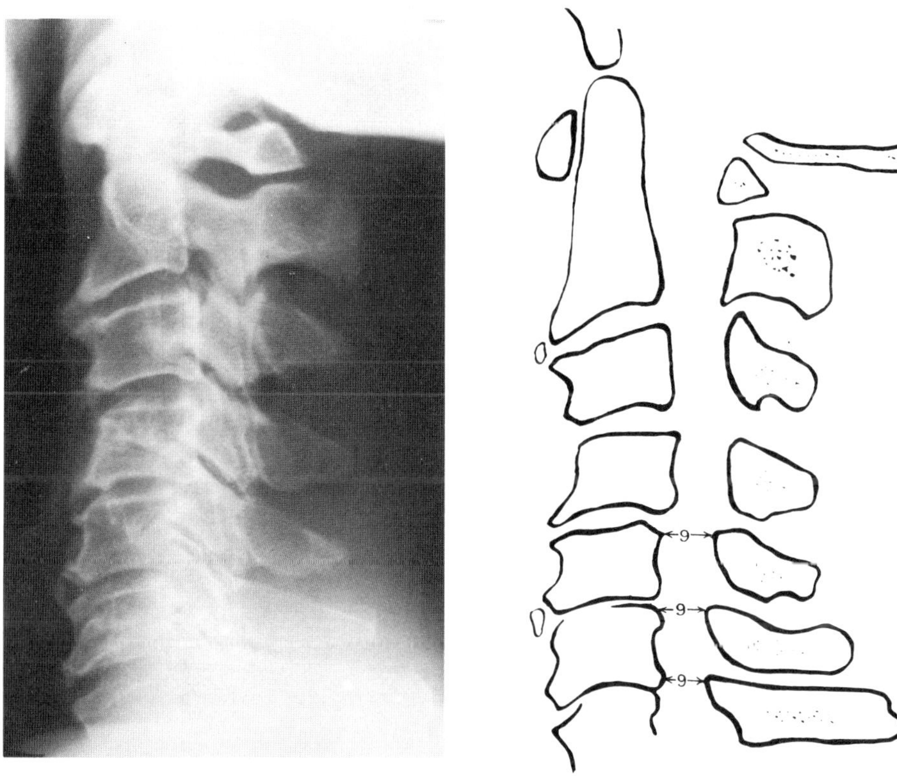

Fig. 8.1 Lateral view of the cervical spine in a case of cervical spondylosis with myelopathy. The canal is generally narrow, measurements in mm between the spurs and the posterior wall of the canal are shown on the trace. (Reproduced with permission from *Neurology*, **17**, 1967)

size of the neural canal at myelography is measured as the distance between the anterior limit of the Myodil column at the level of the maximum indentation of the spondylotic bar, and a point posteriorly at the junction of lamina and spine (Fig. 8.2). This theco-periosteal distance enables measurement in prone myelography where the Myodil will often fail to show the front and back of the neural canal simultaneously. The presence or absence of posterior filling defects due to buckling of the ligamentum flavum is detectable at myelography also (Fig. 8.2), and although this indentation is postero-lateral and not in the midline, it may well represent further embarrassment in an already narrow canal. Theco-periosteal distances of 12 mm or less would be regarded by the present author as essential before the attribution of myelopathic symptoms to cervical spondylosis could be considered. In the majority of cases, a theco-periosteal distance in the region of 10 mm or less will be found at the narrowest point. It is important to note that these measurements are taken directly from X-ray films, with, at

(*a*) (*b*)

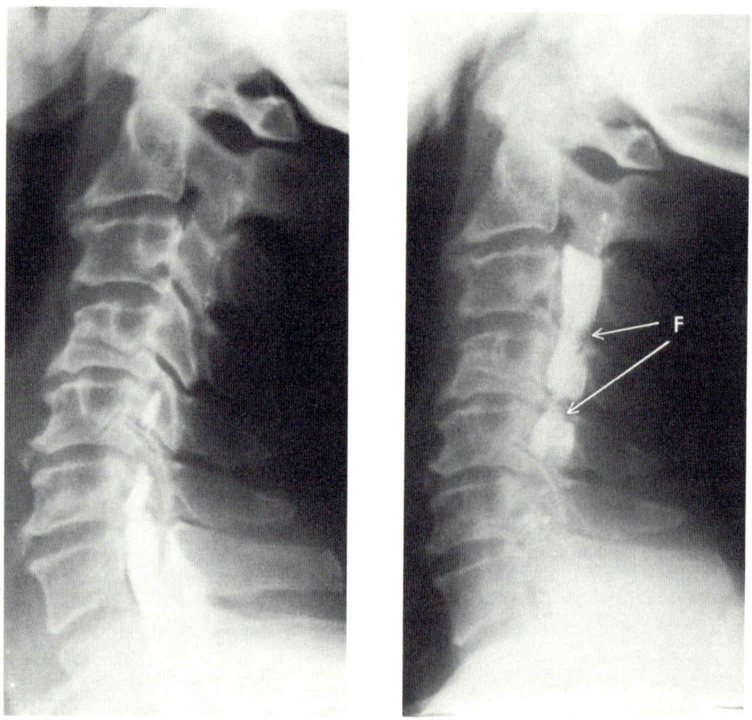

Fig. 8.2 a & b Lateral views of the myelogram in the case whose plain films appear on Fig. 8.1. A tracing of head up and head down screening to show Myodil over the whole constricted area is shown. Posterior indentation from ligamentum flavum appears at several levels (F) and there is considerable obstruction to the Myodil column at C5–6 where the full extent of the narrowing can never be shown. Measurements in mm of the narrowed segment are shown in the trace.
(Reproduced with permission from *Neurology*, **17**, 1967)

myelography, a focus film distance of 54 in. This will mean that myelographic films are slightly more magnified than plain films in which the focus film distance is generally 72 in.

Careful radiology will also indicate whether or not movement is occurring in the spondylotic segment. While some degree of degenerative subluxation is common in cervical spondylosis the presence of exaggerated movement in flexion and extension films is uncommon. It should however be sought for radiologically, since the presence of an appreciably mobile subluxation would prompt the performance of an operation

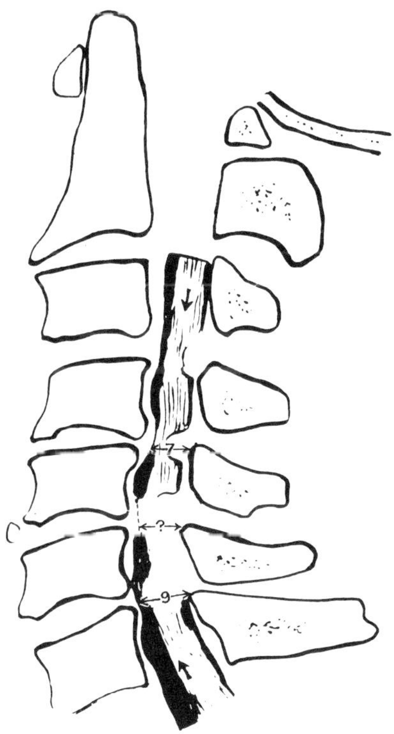

Fig. 8.2c Trace of Fig. 8.2b showing measurement in mm of the narrowed segment

involving fixation at that level rather than a simple decompressive procedure (Fig. 8.3). It is also possible that the presence of cervical kyphosis rather than the more usual lordosis, should prompt caution in the performance of posterior laminectomy.

Provided the criteria described above are fulfilled, operation may be regarded as justified in patients even in advanced age and in poor general condition. Neither the operation of anterior fusion nor of posterior laminectomy as to be described are contra-indicated on the grounds of advanced age. Operation is particularly indicated where progressive deterioration is occurring over a short period of several weeks or months.

It would be of benefit in the assessment of the results of surgery if some standard method of classification could be adopted, possibly the simplest and most generally

(A) (B)

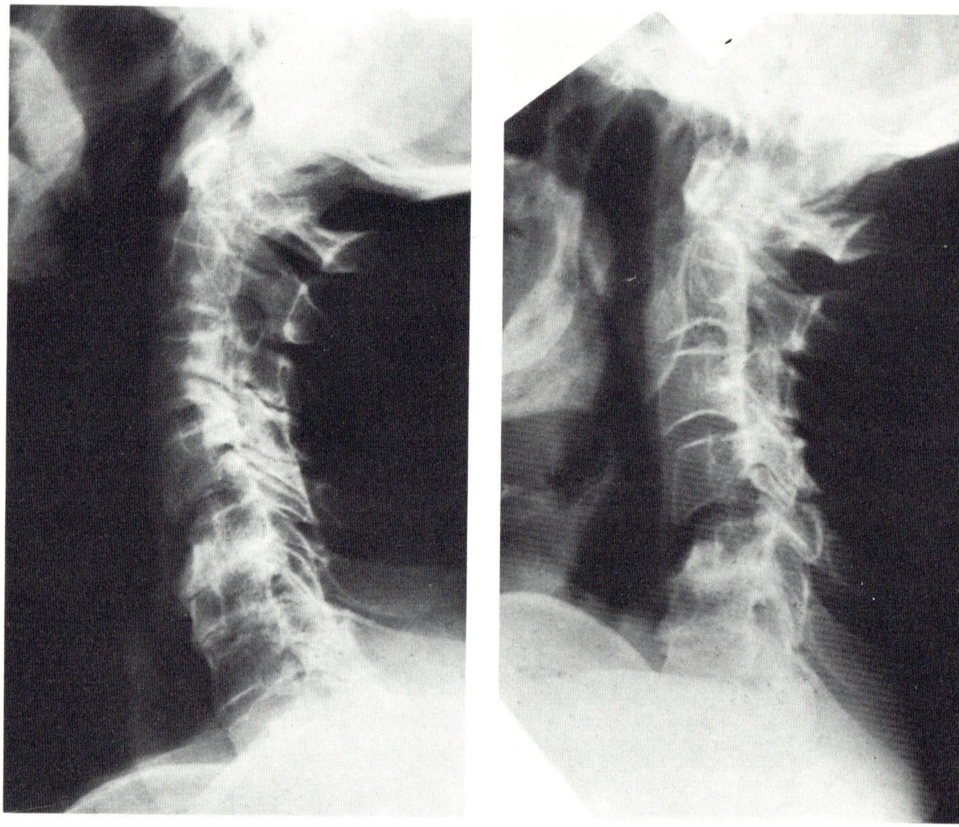

Fig. 8.3 Plain lateral radiographs of the spine in a case of cervical spondylosis with myelopathy. The fixed segment is shown at C5, 6 and 7, but at C4 and C5 forward subluxation is shown on the flexion film (B)

applicable being that of Lees and Aldren Turner (1963) with the addition of a minor modification as suggested by Symon and Lavender (1967). This classification has the merit of simplicity. The grades used are those of mild disability in which the patient though aware of abnormality is not handicapped in his everyday life and, unless other factors are present, is at full time work. Such a grade is as a rule inapplicable as a preoperative assessment since these patients would not be subjected to operation. Moderate disability describes the patient who is appreciably handicapped in his everyday tasks but is partly at work. The grade of severe disability may be divided into two sub-groups; a severe non-bedridden group in which the patient cannot work but is still able to get about indoors, and a severe bedridden group, in which the patient is confined to bed with substantial limb weakness or ataxia, unable to stand or walk unsupported. Operation should be considered in moderate or severe category patients. A rapid deterioration with crossing from one category to another would prompt operation.

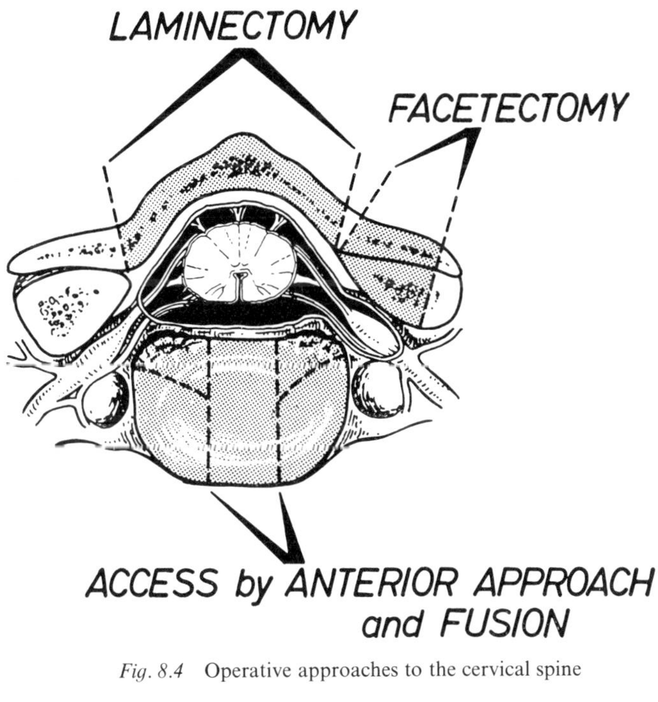

Fig. 8.4 Operative approaches to the cervical spine

Technical Notes on Operations Available in the Treatment of Cervical Spondylosis: The Selection of the Operation for the Patient

As the problems presented to the surgeon by patients with cervical spondylosis differ, so there are different operations which the surgeon may use in their attempted solution. Each operation has its particular merits and drawbacks. It might be supposed that the aim in surgical treatment of cervical spondylosis would be the restoration of normal anatomy in the cervical canal, that is, the removal of spondylotic bars in the canal and in the foramina and the restoration of normal movement at all the intervertebral joints. This ideal it is impossible to achieve. Operations in general have lesser aims. It may be possible in the first place to expand portions of the canal or foramina rendered too narrow by spondylotic spurs (not necessarily by the removal of the spurs themselves, perhaps by the removal of adjacent and more accessible bone) and second, to diminish the irritation of root structures or the formation of osteophytes by reducing the movement between contiguous vertebral bodies through fusion procedures. Decompression operations involve removal of laminae (laminectomy), or portions of the intervertebral foramina (foraminotomy, facetectomy), or both, and are undertaken from a posterior approach (Fig. 8.4). Fusion procedures now commonly employed involve removal of the disc and adjacent bone together perhaps with accessible spurs in the vertebral canal and foramina, and subsequent fusion by bone graft between vertebral bodies. They are undertaken from the anterior approach. Posterior fusion techniques are now less commonly employed.

Indications for and performance of anterior fusion operations

Where cervical spinal disease can be strictly localised to one intervertebral level and where the sagittal diameter of the remainder of the canal is normal, the operation of choice can now be seen to be anterior fusion by any of the commonly available methods. Such cases arise particularly many years after trauma but form on the whole a small minority of patients presenting either with the radicular or myelopathic features of spondylosis. However, where the spondylotic changes are localised to one space whether the patient suffers from myelopathy or radiculopathy, then anterior fusion is the operation of choice.

In the patient with a spinal canal of normal width, where the changes are limited to two adjacent intervertebral disc spaces, the anterior fusion operation would still be the choice of many surgeons. It would be the author's view that if the needs for operation were dictated by root compression then under these circumstances anterior fusion would be preferred. The choice of operation for a two level spondylosis with myelopathic features is dependent upon certain other factors. Amongst these would be the presence or absence of movement in flexion and extension at the pathological joints and particularly upon evidence of abnormal movement at joints apart from the spondylotic area. If movement persists in the spondylotic segment, unassociated with an abnormal range of movement elsewhere and the diameter of the remainder of the canal is within normal limits, anterior fusion would still seem to be indicated. More commonly, however, two level spondylosis shows little movement at the affected joints, commonly the three vertebrae involved form a fairly rigid segment with overlapping of the laminae and a considerable lordosis, the "shingling" referred to by Crandall and Batzdorf (1966), and under these circumstances a decompressive procedure from behind would seem to be best. Where the adjacent joints show evidence of excessive movement then the risks of throwing further strain upon these joints by further fixation of the spondylotic segment, would weigh against the use of an anterior fusion procedure. Then with multiple levels involved, particularly in the presence of a congenitally narrow canal, the anterior operation is unsuitable either for radiculopathy or myelopathy.

The Performance of the Anterior Operation

The technical details of anterior interbody fusion are excellently described in a number of publications by Smith and Robinson (1958) and Cloward (1963). The neck, slightly extended and rotated a little to the left, is supported upon a sandbag. A skin crease incision is used, its level in the neck dependent upon the cervical intervertebral space to be reached, as a general rule an incision in the region of the cricoid is suitable for the C6–7 or 5–6 levels, this incision or one at the level of the lower third of the thyroid cartilage for C4–5, and a rather higher incision for the most difficult space to reach by this manoeuvre, C3–4. The plane of cleavage between the sternomastoid and the paratracheal musculature is developed, and dissection pursued between the carotid sheath laterally and the trachea and oesophagus medially. Both these groups of structures are readily dissected by gauze dissection of the cervical fascia to expose the anterior aspect of the cervical spine with its covering musculature. At this point, plain lateral films of the neck should be taken with a needle or other marker in the disc space so that certain identification of the disc space is obtained. In the Smith and Robinson procedure, the disc is then removed piecemeal, skull or halter traction used to separate the vertebral bodies, and fusion performed with a block of iliac bone. Spurs are not removed from the foramina and spinal canal in this procedure. In the Cloward technique which is the author's personal preference, the disc and the contiguous portions of the vertebral bodies are drilled out by special drills, and curettes used to remove the spurs from the canal and from the intervertebral foramina. There is some evidence that in the treatment of radiculopathy, dissection of the intervertebral disc down to the level of the dura is unnecessary, since sound fusion of the intervertebral spaces has been alleged to produce resorption of osteophytes within the intervertebral foramina. It is the author's practice, however, to remove these spurs as far as possible, a procedure which involves the dissection of the intervertebral disc space to the level of the dura in order to obtain adequate identification of the landmarks, but it is certain that complete removal of the spurs is impossible by any manoeuvre. Fusion of the vertebral bodies may be performed by the insertion of a dowel cut from the iliac crest, by the insertion of prepared ox-bone (Kiel bone) or by the insertion of a tibial cortical graft as preferred by Verbiest and Paz Y Geuse (1968). Of these the simplest is the iliac or Kiel bone dowel.

An antero-lateral approach to the intervertebral foramina or the vertebral artery using a modification of the Henry (1966) technique, has recently been re-described by Verbiest and it may be that this operation will prove as satisfactory for laterally placed intervertebral spurs as for the unusual cases of compression of the vertebral artery from spurs in the intervertebral foramen.

Disadvantages and Dangers of the Anterior Procedure

The anterior procedure involves dissection towards the cervical spinal canal through a block of bone and the final stages of removal of osteophytes from the vertebral canal or from the intervertebral foramina must be performed with considerable care. Damage to the cord with a post-operative worsening of the myelopathic symptoms, or to the roots, has been recorded, but with increasing familiarity with the operation and a reasonable standard of operative skill, there is no doubt that this is a straightforward and safe procedure.

Less certain, however, is the effect which the fusion, particularly of several levels, may have upon the biomechanics of the cervical spine. The development of accelerated degeneration at adjacent intervertebral levels has been recorded by a number of authors, and increased stress must be thrown upon the adjacent discs with fusion of one of their number. In one personal case, where anterior interbody fusion was performed for an acute soft prolapse of a cervical disc with paraparesis, not in a spondylotic spine, degeneration and prolapse of the disc below followed within twelve months by a recurrence of symptoms, necessitating further surgery to the lower level.

The operation presents its greatest applicability at the levels C4–5, 5–6 or 6–7. It can be difficult to perform at C3–4 and its difficulties are maximal in the patient with a short thick neck. Lesser complications of the anterior procedure are transient dysphagia and hoarseness from retraction of the pharynx and larynx and troublesome wound haematomas.

In a certain proportion of cases, fusion fails to take place. The incidence of this is failure variously given as 21 per cent (Connolly *et al.*, 1965), 2 per cent (Cloward, 1963), 5 per cent (Stuck *et al.*, 1960), 26 per cent (Dereymaeker and Mulier, 1958), 1 per cent (Herzberger *et al.*, 1962). There is some disagreement as to the correlation between the adequacy of fusion and the clinical result. Thus Dereymaeker and Mulier felt that their results were directly related to the adequacy of the fusion and a similar view was expressed by Herzberger *et al.* (1963). Robinson *et al.* (1962), on the other hand, could not correlate the adequacy of fusion with the clinical result.

Posterior approaches to the cervical spine

(a) Foraminotomy for radiculopathy

In patients with radiculopathy from cervical spondylosis, filling defects may be detectable on the myelogram laterally placed in the foramina at many levels. Where more than one nerve root is clearly involved clinically, or where the distribution of the nerve roots clinically cannot be fitted accurately into one level, it may be difficult to plan an adequate operation by the anterior route. Where more than two intervertebral foramina have to be decompressed, it has been the author's practice to perform foraminotomy from the posterior approach. The technique of operation has been described by Frykholm (1947) and its first stages are essentially similar to those of laminectomy, the spines and laminae of the appropriate vertebrae being cleared from a posterior midline incision. Surgery for radiculopathy is commonly carried out on one side and only unilateral stripping of the spines and laminae need be performed. The intervertebral foramen is best opened into well laterally, and a useful technique is to use a rose burr to develop the approach to the posterior part of the foramen with the spines and laminae intact. A power tool such as the Hall drill is useful for this purpose also. The dissection is carried out into the lateral mass enlarging the foramen and gently dissecting flakes of bone from the surface of the root with fine instruments after the bone has been thinned down by the power drill. The final exposure reveals the lateral third of the theca, together with the emergent root in its dural sheath. Frykholm emphasised further the necessity for division of the dural sheath and of any septa between the nerve roots, but this modification of the procedure is not commonly employed. The lateral extent of the foraminotomy should be beyond any palpable spurs within the intervertebral foramen although removal of these spurs anterior to the root will depend upon local conditions at the time of operation. Foraminotomy by this technique may be employed for three or four levels at one time.

Where foraminotomy has been performed at multiple levels, some interference with the stability of the spine may be expected and post-operative immobilisation will be necessary. As compared with the anterior procedure for radiculopathy, the patient is in considerably greater discomfort post-operatively and since the operation carries no component of fusion, it is less likely to prevent progression of the condition.

(b) Laminectomy for the myelopathy of cervical spondylosis

The posterior approach is indicated primarily in patients where the cervical lordosis is exaggerated, overlap of laminae is detectable at multiple levels on the plain films, there is extensive narrowing of the cervical canal on a congenital basis, and multiple levels of spondylotic narrowing present in the anterior aspect of the canal. An additional indication is severe limitation of movement of the cervical spine so that instability does not appear to be a factor in progression of the condition.

The operation is best performed under general anaesthesia in the prone position, and particular care is necessary to prevent hyper-extension of the neck at any stage either during the initiation of anaesthetic and intubation, or during the positioning of the patient on the table. With a narrow canal and multiple spondylotic bars, the spinal cord is at particular risk during extension. Numerous examples of deterioration of patients with hitherto unsuspected cervical spondylosis, have occurred in the author's experience following general anaesthesia for some other quite unassociated condition such as an abdominal operation, and it seems likely that the factor here has been extension of the neck during intubation. The spine is approached by a midline incision from the exion to the spine of the vertebra prominens, and the spines and laminae of as many vertebrae as would appear to be involved in the canal narrowing, exposed. It is preferable to leave the muscular attachments to C2 if at all possible, as extensive dissection of the muscular attachments over the entire cervical spine may result in increasing kyphosis post-operatively. The importance of strong musculature in the post-operative period has been stressed by a number of authors, particularly Aboulker

(1956). It is usually necessary to remove the spines and laminae of vertebrae above and below the offending disc space, and in such patients a common laminectomy would involve C3, 4, 5 and 6. Removal of the upper border of C3 without the complete dissection of the musculature from C2 may prove tedious, but it is not impracticable. Great care is necessary in the performance of the laminectomy, since there is frequently very little room between the lamina and dura, while the subarachnoid space posteriorly is almost obliterated so that the cord is not as usual protected by a cushion of c.s.f. from manipulation of the laminae. The blades of instruments should never be introduced beneath the laminae, which should be scaled off by meticulous dissection from the back. The laminectomy should be carried out to the lateral margin of the canal so that a blunt hook may be introduced forwards at the level of the pedicles without lateral deviation. The ligamentum flavum is removed from the entire length of the bone involved in the laminectomy. There are differing opinions as to the wisdom or necessity for opening the dura. Neither opening of the dura nor division of the dentate ligaments (Kahn, 1947) are commonly practised, since they involve further manipulation in the region of an already damaged spinal cord, although evidence has recently been presented (Crandall and Batzdorf, 1966) to suggest that a linear incision of the dura with repair by the insertion of an elliptical graft of neodura, may have some merit.

If it is desired to open up intervertebral foramina, the technique of foraminotomy mentioned briefly in the previous paragraph should be performed before the laminectomy is begun, since it is considerably easier with the laminae intact.

Following laminectomy for cervical spondylosis, provided the cervical spine is rigid, and no more than three laminae have been removed, it is not necessary to perform post-operative immobilisation, although exercises to the cervical spine are stressed in particular by Aboulker (1956). Where more than four laminae have been removed or where the operation has been combined with facetectomy, some form of post-operative support is necessary. A firm metal reinforced collar supporting the chin upon the shoulders is usually adequate although immobilisation by Crutchfield calipers with 10 lb traction for 2 weeks (Northfield and Osmond-Clarke, 1967) has been recommended.

(c) Posterior fusion operations

The operation of posterior fusion by the application of onlay grafts after rawing the laminae using cortical bone from the iliac crest and iliac bone chips has been largely superseded by techniques of anterior fusion. It was an operation which required a considerable period of immobilisation either in a plaster bed or in a Minerva plaster and which was therefore unsuitable for patients with advanced myelopathy.

Disadvantages and Dangers of the Posterior Operation

In the hands of a skilled surgeon laminectomy even in patients of advanced age and poor general condition should be an operation with a low mortality.

If the operation is performed in the seated position, the hazard of air embolus is ever present, but this is avoided by the use of the prone position, with or without assisted respiration. Even in careful hands, however, there is some risk of damage to the cervical cord which in advanced myelopathy is thinned and already embarrassed by the presence of ischaemic changes. Complete transection with quadriparesis has occasionally occurred after laminectomy. Careful attention to operative detail, and to the avoidance of hyper-extension during intubation will reduce such disastrous complications to minimum levels, certainly under 1 per cent.

A more serious criticism of the posterior operation for myelopathy is that the basic pathology, degeneration of the discs and the development of spurs in the anterior portion of the canal, is left unchanged. Attempts have indeed been made to remove spurs by the posterior approach, but because of the extreme fragility of the cervical cord already referred to, these have been attended by increased incidence of deterioration sometimes of disastrous degree, and are probably unjustified.

Operations for compression of the vertebral artery

Compression of the vertebral artery has been reported (Hardin, 1960; Gortvai, 1964; Brain, 1963; Sheehan *et al.*, 1960) in association with cervical spondylosis. Vertebral angiography will be necessary to confirm the presence of a localised compression of the vertebral artery at the level of one or more interspaces, and it is necessary to perform angiography with full lateral rotation (Sheehan and Meyer, 1960; Maslowski, 1960; Hardin, 1960), since the maximal compression of the artery may occur only in a position of full rotation. It is, however, particularly difficult to decide the part played by such spondylotic compression, since vertebro-basilar ischaemia occurs in patients with, as a rule, considerable atheromatous change elsewhere in the basilar circulation so that the part played by the spondylotic spur is frequently open to doubt.

If, however, it seems desirable to remove the spurs to decompress the vertebral artery, this is best performed by the antero-lateral approach as described in detail by Verbiest (1968).

The results of surgical treatment of cervical spondylosis

Assessment of the results of surgical treatment of cervical spondylosis, as indeed of the results of medical treatment of the condition, are bedevilled by the lack of uniformity of clinical description in the various published reports. Two of the principal causes have been that the results of surgery are frequently presented so that it is impossible to differentiate data relating to radiculopathy from that relating to myelopathy. The two conditions frequently require a different operative approach, and their spontaneous prognosis is quite different, so that in discussion of the results of surgical treatment it is essential to separate the two. A further source of confusion has been that published series claiming to represent surgery for cervical spondylosis especially with radicular symptoms, have frequently included surgery for acute prolapse of the cervical intervertebral discs. This is a condition which has a differing age group, is very much more localised, and presents as a rule in a different way, although, as in every other field of clinical medicine, it may require considerable diagnostic thought to distinguish a sub-acute presentation of soft disc prolapse in a middle-aged patient from the fairly rapid development of cervical spondylosis; the clinical picture and the age group of both may clearly overlap. In presentation of results, however, separation between the two is essential, as the recent literature bears out.

Comparison of the results of surgery by the various approaches is even more difficult since large series of anterior fusions, particularly for myelopathy, have not to date been reported.

TABLE 8.1 *Results of operation for root compression*

	Improved	*Unchanged or worse*	*Total no. of cases*
(a) *By the posterior approach*			
Frykholm (1951)	25	5	30
Spurling (1956)	55	6	61
Haft and Shenkin (1963)	27	2	29
Knight (1964)	22	3	25
Totals	129 (89%)	16 (11%)	145
(b) *By the anterior approach*			
Connolly *et al.* (1965)	24	13	37
Verbiest and Paz Y Geuse (1966)	26	1	27
Galera and Tovi (1968)	14	4	18
Totals	64 (78%)	18 (22%)	82

A list of published results for the treatment of radiculopathy is given in Table 8.1. The groups reported before 1960 were by the posterior approach where the surgery to the root pathology was that of facetectomy or foraminotomy. While the statistics appear almost uniformly encouraging, the wide variation in the severity of the condition for which operation was performed, and the before mentioned variation in the criteria for assessment (with the inclusion of data relating to soft disc) make strict comparison difficult. It is the author's view, however, from his own and his colleague's experience, that the results of foraminotomy for the radiculopathy of cervical spondylosis are not as encouraging as published series would lead one to suppose, although a worthwhile improvement may be obtained in about 60 per cent of patients.

It seems likely, although as yet no firm conclusion could be made, that the results of the anterior fusion operation are rather superior. Thus even in a fairly discouraging review of the treatment of cervical spondylosis as a whole by anterior disc excision by Galera and Tovi (1968) in Sweden, worthwhile results were obtained in nearly 80 per cent of cases of radiculopathy. Criteria for selection involved operation in only one or two levels in 18 cases.

It would be the author's view that anterior interbody fusion at one or two levels is the operation of choice provided the patient does not have a congenitally narrow canal.

The results of the surgical treatment of spondylotic myelopathy are rather more extensively documented, since the operation principally practiced for this condition, posterior laminectomy, has been employed and reported for over 20 years. A summary of the results is appended in Table 8.2. It seems clear that between 60 and 70 per cent

TABLE 8.2 *Results of operation for myelopathy*

	Improved	*Unchanged*	*Worse*	*Total no. of cases*
(a) *By the posterior approach*				
Northfield (1955)	22	8	8	38
Clarke and Robinson (1956)	13	4	14	31
Guidetti (1961)	48	10	6	64
Peserico *et al* (1962)	18	26	3	47
Harris (1965)	20	6	8	34
Stoops and King (1965)	35	7	0	42
Crandall and Batzdorf (1966)	16	7	11	34
Symon and Lavender (1967)	29	9	2	40
Totals	201 (61%)	77 (23%)	52 (16%)	330
(b) *By the anterior approach*				
Crandall and Batzdorf (1966)	15	2	4	21
Verbiest and Paz Y Geuse (1966)	7	2	0	9
Galera and Tovi (1968)	3	9	0	12
Totals	25 (60%)	13 (31%)	4 (9%)	42

of patients subjected to a laminectomy for the criteria mentioned in the present chapter will show some improvement. The results however are not likely to be as striking as the disappearance of pain in the radiculopathic case, but they are beyond doubt worth while. Thus in the surgical series reviewed by Symon and Lavender (1967), of 25 cases falling into the pre-operative category of severe disablement, 60 per cent improved at least to the extent of being able to get out of the house and do some shopping having previously been confined to house or bed; 24 per cent improved by two of the clinical categories used in assessment from severe to mild disability, and it is worth stressing that this last figure represents patients who, having been confined to their house or bed due to a combination of spasticity and ataxia or both, have been able to return to work or normal activity with no serious disability remaining. In common with the experience of others the greatest improvement has often occurred in the old, the frail and the bed-bound, particularly where the progression from ambulation to confinement to bed has been rapid.

Some evidence of a permanent influence of surgery was pointed out by Symon and Lavender from alterations in the clinical pattern of the disease post-operatively. Cervical spondylosis may show a continuous and progressive deterioration, or, not infrequently, a course of spontaneous remission and subsequent relapse often on several occasions over many years. In cases with a progressive history, the advent of improvement following surgery might be regarded as coincidental with the advent of a natural remission. Thirty-two of forty-eight of Symon and Lavender's patients showed a progressive history, two becoming worse after operation and 30 either remaining static or improving, at any rate their continuous deterioration being arrested. Sixteen patients however presented clear evidence of remission in the previous history, many having had conservative treatment during relapse. Over a follow-up extending to at least 2 years, only two patients had a further relapse and one must presume that in the majority of this group, therefore, the disease had been appreciably modified by surgery. It is clear, however, that only a very prolonged follow-up of such cases will enable further refinement of the choice for or against surgery and of the various types of surgery to be made on logical grounds.

Comparison of medical and surgical series is also difficult and probably not worth while. In this country at any rate, the usual practice is to persist in medical treatment until the disability becomes at least moderate in extent but once this stage has been reached, comparison of figures where possible (Symon and Lavender) suggests that laminectomy has appreciably better results than persistence in conservative treatment.

References

Aboulker, J., Metzger, J., David, M., Engel, P. and Ballivet, J. (1956), *Neurochirurgie*, **11**, 87.
Brain, W. R. (1963), *Brit. med. J.*, **1**, 771.
Burrows, E. H. (1963), *Clin. Radiol.*, **14**, 77.
Cloward, R. B. (1958), *J. Neurosurg.*, **15**, 602.
Cloward, R. B. (1963), *Clin. Orthoped.*, **27**, 51.
Connolly, E. S., Seymour, R. J. and Adams, J. E. (1965), *J. Neurosurg.*, **23**, 431.
Crandall, P. H. and Batzdorf, U. (1966), *J. Neurosurg.*, **25**, 57.
Dereymaeker, A. and Mulier, J. (1958), *Rev. Neurol.*, **99**, 597.
Frykholm, R. (1947), *Acta. Chir. Scand.*, suppl. 160.
Galera, R. and Tovi, D. (1968), *J. Neurosurg.*, **28**, 305.
Gortvai, P. (1964), *Brit. med. J.*, **2**, 233.
Hardin, C. A., Williamson, W. P. and Steegmann, A. T. (1960), *Neurology*, **10**, 855.
Henry, A. K. (1966), *Extensile Exposure*, E. & S. Livingstone, Edinburgh and London, p. 58.
Hertzberger, E. E., Chandler, A., Bear, N. E. and Kindschi, L. G. (1962), *Clin. Orthoped.*, **24**, 83.
Hertzberger, E. E., Kindschi, L. G., Bear, N. E. and Chandler, A. (1963), *Neurochir.*, **23**, 215.
Kahn, E. A. (1947), *J. Neurosurg.*, **4**, 191.
Kuhlendahl, H. and Kunert, W. (1954), *Die Medisinische*, **14**, 449.
Lees, F. and Turner, J. W. A. (1963), *Brit. med. J.*, **2**, 1607.
Mair, W. G. P. and Druckman, R. (1953), *Brain*, **76**, 70.
Maslowski, H. A. (1960), *J. Neurol. Neurosurg. and Psychiat.*, **23**, 355.
Northfield, D. W. C. and Osmond-Clarke, H. (1967), *Cervical Spondylosis*, ed Brain and Wilkinson, 1st edn., Heineman,, p. 207.
Pallis, C., Jones, A. M. and Spillane, J. D. (1954), *Brain*, **77**, 274.
Robinson, R. A. and Smith, G. W. (1955), *Bull John's Hopkins Hosp.*, **96**, 223.

Robinson, R. A., Walker, A. E., Farlic, D. C. and Wiecking, D. K. (1962), *J. Bone Jt. Surg.*, **44a**, 1569.
Sheehan, S., Bauer, R. B. and Meyer, J. S. (1960), *Neurology*, **10**, 968.
Smith, G. W. and Robinson, R. A. (1958), *J. Bone Jt. Surg.*, **40a**, 607.
Stuck, R. M., Hall, R. F. and Fralick, E. H. (1960), *Amer. Surgeon*, **26**, 50.
Symon, L. and Lavender, P. (1967), *Neurology*, **17**, 117.
Taylor, A. R. (1964), *Neurology*, **14**, 62.
Verbiest, H. and Paz Y Geuse, H. D. (1966), *J. Neurosurg.*, **25**, 611.
Verbiest, H. (1968), *J. Neurosurg.*, **28**, 191.
Wolf, B. S., Khilnani, M. and Mallus, L. (1956), *J. Mount Sinai Hosp.*, **23**, 283.

Chapter IX

Prognosis

MARCIA WILKINSON

General Considerations

A study of the pathology of the nerve roots and spinal cord in cervical spondylosis shows how complex may be the factors causing damage. Pressure, ischaemia, fibrosis of nerve-roots, neuronal degeneration in nerve-roots and spinal cord, oedema in both situations, and the effects of neck movement—any or all of these may play a part in each case. Some of these changes must be reversible or improvement would not occur with medical treatment only; others such as nerve cell destruction will not improve whatever the treatment. The available statistics of prognosis are discussed below, but generalisations apply to the individual patient to only a limited extent. It is necessary to assess as far as possible the individual factors operating in the production of symptoms in order to arrive at the prognosis for any particular patient.

RADICULOPATHY

In acute radiculopathy there appears to be a natural tendency to improvement. This has been brought out by the trial arranged by the British Association of Physical Medicine (1966) into the effects of different types of treatment on pain in the neck and arms. The Committee responsible for the investigation began by defining "a symptom-complex", this trial being designed to assess the effects of different types of treatment on patients with "pain in the neck and arm". The patients selected had to comply with one of the following sets of criteria:

(a) Pain in the neck and arm with or without paraesthesiae, the symptoms having a root distribution and being associated with limited and painful movements of the neck.
(b) Pain in the neck and arm of full root distribution with paraesthesiae but without clinical evidence of abnormality in the neck.
(c) Pain or paraesthesiae in the neck and arm of partial root distribution but with definite evidence of clinical abnormality in the neck.

Unfortunately in this trial no effort was made to assess the degree of involvement of any particular nerve root or roots, nor was the presence of any abnormalities in the nervous system such as diminution or absence of reflexes, or sensory loss recorded. Patients in whom the symptoms were apparently due solely to local lesions, such as cervical rib, rotator cuff lesions of the shoulder, tennis elbow or carpal tunnel syndrome were excluded, as were those with abnormal neurological signs indicating cord compression and those who had definitive disorders of the cervical spine such as rheumatoid arthritis or Paget's disease, or who had had a bony injury to the cervical spine in the preceding 12 months.

The patients were allotted to 5 treatment groups in a random fashion, as follows.

Group I—had aspirin, instruction in posture, a collar and traction.
Group II—had the same treatment except that the patient was put in a position that gave maximum relief of pain but no traction was applied.
Group III—had aspirin, instruction in posture and a collar.
Group IV—had placebo (heat); aspirin and untuned short-wave diathermy.
Group V—had placebo (inert tablets); and aspirin taken three times a day.

This trial suffered from the serious defect that it was based upon the treatment of a symptom-complex without adequate assessment of its cause. Nevertheless, the data suggest that a considerable proportion of the patients were suffering from radiculopathy secondary to cervical spondylosis, and it was found that the rate of improvement was approximately the same in the five treatment groups as judged by clinical assessment 2 weeks and 4 weeks after the beginning of treatment, and by follow-up questionnaire at 6 weeks and 6 months. The degree of improvement at 4 weeks was however influenced by age, the initial severity of symptoms, the number of previous attacks, the duration of previous attacks, and whether the patient was getting better or worse when first seen.

Thus there would seem to be a natural tendency for the pain of radiculopathy to improve considerably in a period of from 4 to 6 weeks from the onset. It would not, however, appear justifiable to draw conclusions as to the value of particular forms of treatment from a mass investigation of this kind, which does not include an attempt to make an assessment of the precise nature and extent of the lesion being treated. Some patients while losing their pain continue to suffer indefinitely from tingling sensations and impairment of cutaneous sensibility in their fingers.

Recurrence of the symptoms is not uncommon and may occur after a few months or after many years. Sometimes a new attack occurs on the same, and sometimes on the opposite side, the site of the symptoms depending on the root or roots involved.

In an acute radiculopathy with severe muscular weakness and wasting of radicular distribution the prognosis is usually good and there is likely to be a substantial recovery of power, though this may take as long as 2 years.

MYELOPATHY

Once the signs and symptoms of myelopathy have occurred it is rare for the signs to regress and any improvement is usually subjective. With treatment there is often an initial improvement which may be due partly to psychological factors but very often this is followed later by deterioration.

Brain, Northfield and Wilkinson (1962) thought that the prognosis was adversely affected by age, severe cord damage, multiple disc lesions, and a long history, and considered that if operation were to be done it was most likely to be successful in those who had a short history of cord signs. Clarke and Robinson (1964) felt that the prognosis was independent of age, the duration of symptoms or the severity of the anatomical change in the cervical spine. Lees and Turner (1963) thought that the age of onset and the severity of the clinical picture were important, while Bradshaw (1957) suggested that there was a mild form of spondylotic myelopathy in which arrest of progress occurred independently of any treatment given. James (1965) thought that the prognosis was independent of age, sex, trauma, a history of degenerative changes in the spine, the dimensions of the spinal canal, type of clinical picture and extent of initial disability, but that it was adversely affected with the duration of symptoms before diagnosis, and the increase of protein in the cerebrospinal fluid. He also commented on the overall similarity of results in patients treated medically and surgically. He explained these facts by the hypothesis that there are two types of change in the cervical cord, an acute "exudative" and partially reversible condition, and a process of gradual loss of neuronal tissue with consequent demyelination and gliosis. The factor which prevents the former from progressing inevitably to the latter may well be the development of an adequate collateral circulation. Symon and Lavender (1967) consider that between 60 and 70 per cent of patients subjected to laminectomy show some improvement, to the extent of being able to get out of the house to do some shopping having previously been confined to the house or bed. They also think that the relapse rate is lower in those who have had a laminectomy and that operation should be done as soon as the disability becomes moderate and that delay may prejudice the results of surgery.

These conflicting views show how hard it is to draw conclusions from existing data. The usual course of the disorder seems to be that the average patient with cervical myelopathy deteriorates slowly over a period of a year or two, after which the symptoms may remain stationary for a long time. Often, therefore, cervical myelopathy is virtually a self-limiting disorder. Pathologically, one may perhaps look upon the phase of deterioration as the result of recurrent trauma to which the spinal cord eventually adapts itself if the narrowing of the canal is not progressive. There are two exceptions, both involving a minority of patients. The course may from the beginning be more acute, and progressive deterioration occur in spite of treatment. Or, again, though the course is not more rapid, the usual fairly complete arrest does not occur and progressive deterioration continues, again in spite of treatment. It is in these two rarer groups of cases that one sees a terminal paraplegia or quadriplegia with loss of sphincter control, and these are the patients most likely to benefit from early operation. The length of the history before treatment and immediate response to treatment are the best guides to prognosis. The indication for and the prognosis after surgery have been discussed in Chapter VIII. As already pointed out, trauma is likely to cause a deterioration in cervical myelopathy much of which may be irreversible.

When cervical spondylosis was first recognised as a cause of myelopathy it appeared to fall into the category of extramedullary compression of the spinal cord calling for surgical intervention. Later knowledge of the complexity of the pathology led to a more conservative attitude to surgery simply for the relief of the myelopathy.

The large number of patients treated surgically and the different standards of selection of patients for operation has made it hard to assess prognosis of the myelopathy in cases treated medically, and hence, incidentally, the indications for surgery. The figures of the various series are capable of more than one interpretation since we do not know accurately what would have happened to the patients if they had been treated medically rather than surgically. Nevertheless following surgery some patients have shown a quite dramatic improvement, beyond that which could have been expected to occur spontaneously.

References

Bradshaw, P. (1957), *Quart. J. Med.*, **26**, 177.
Brain, W. R., Northfield, D. W. C. and Wilkinson, M. (1952), *Brain*, **75**, 187.
British Association of Physical Medicine (1966), *Brit. med. J.*, **1**, 253.
Clarke, E. and Robinson, P. K. (1956), *Brain*, **79**, 483.
James, J. L. (1965), "The Treatment of Myelopathy due to Cervical Spondylosis", M.D. Thesis, Bristol University.
Lees, F. and Turner, J. W. A. (1963), *Brit. med. J.*, **2**, 1607.
Symon, L. and Lavender, P. (1967), *Neurology*, **17**, 117.

Index